GOOD CHILDBIRTH

*How to have the pregnancy
and childbirth you deserve*

by

DR STEVEN REID

FOREWORD

by

PROFESSOR WENDY SAVAGE

GOOD CHILDBIRTH

© 1999 Dr Steven Reid

The right of Dr Steven Reid to be identified as the author of this work has been asserted by him in accordance with the Copyright, Designs and Patents Act 1988

All rights reserved. No part of this publication may be reproduced, stored in a retrieval system, or transmitted in any form or by any means, electronic, mechanical, photocopying, recording or otherwise, without the prior permission of the author.

ISBN 0 9535011 0 8

First published in 1999 in a limited edition of three-thousand copies of which this copy is number

Typeset and printed by BDP Design and Print of Chorley

Published and distributed by Rosses Publications,
10 Ansdell Road North, Lytham, Lancashire, England

FOREWORD

by
Professor Wendy Savage

I would thoroughly recommend this book to pregnant women who want to have as good an experience in labour and as natural a birth as possible.

Dr Reid has used language in his own particular way to get his message across - although I would not describe a woman having the misfortune to vomit in pregnancy as a 'puker' I can nevertheless understand just what he means!

His ideas are extremely interesting and provocative.

This work is a useful addition to the literature about childbirth.

Wendy Savage

Good Childbirth

By giving birth

You extend the boundaries of the Universe

Into Eternity

You write your name in heaven

You take part in Creation

Source unknown

DEDICATION

To my wife Mary

and all the other expectant mothers

who taught me far more

about the mystery and miracle of childbirth

than I ever taught them

PREFACE

My eldest daughter is coming up to her GCSE's and therefore brings with her opinions the certainty of youth. When she casually scanned the draft of a chapter of this book, she proclaimed: "Dad, this English is rubbish." I cheerfully agreed with her.

The ideal way for you to absorb the ideas put forward in 'GOOD CHILDBIRTH' would be for me to give you my thoughts at the same time that you gave me yours. To present them in book form is unavoidably onesided. To minimise this weakness, I have set down my thoughts as I would say them to you.

So the English is rubbish. Many sentences start with 'but' or 'and'. There's lots of repetition. For this I make no apology. If as you read it, you can begin to feel the sense behind what I am saying, then you will gain the benefit.

At times I might be using 'you', 'we' and 'I' in the same paragraph when I am trying to get an idea across. It might seem confusing at first, but bear with me and read it over again. You'll soon begin to feel why I have presented the message in that way.

Don't worry if you have to keep on coming back to 'have another go' at some sections. Absorb them in any order you like. It's all down to what you find works for you. As you will find out, there's more than one 'you' and you might find it takes a little time before the 'you' that matters gets into the ideas that I am presenting.

And at the end of the day I hope you will have the pregnancy and labour you deserve.

Contents

1. Where do we begin? 1
2. Where have we gone wrong? 5
3. How we start off on the wrong foot. 11
4. A good labour or a lousy labour - what's the difference? 27
5. How do I get the labour I want? 41
6. Let's clear the decks 51
7. Puking 65
8. Intermission 77
9. So where do you fancy going? 85
10. The big day 93
11. What if my labour isn't normal ? 101
12. Have we got an attitude problem? 113
13. Options you have for your labour 121
14. The way forward 129
15. So how was it for you? 139

Acknowledgements

Thanks are due to Professor Wendy Savage for her helpful advice, thoughtful comments and foreword.

The illustration on the front cover is by Eleanor Drage of Loughborough High School.

The illustration on the back cover is by Matthew Pickering of Arnold School Blackpool

The illustrations on pages sixty-eight and eighty-two are by Tim Hatton of Arnold School Blackpool.

The illustrations on pages thirty-three, thirty-five, fifty-five and sixty-three were designed by Paul Cardwell.

The photographs of the interior of the Chapel of the Rotunda Hospital were taken by the author with the permission of the Master of the Hospital.

Chapter One

Where do we Begin?

15th March 1745 was a momentous day in the history of the care of women in childbirth. It was on that day that the doors opened of the first maternity hospital in the British Isles, the Dublin Hospital for Poor Lying-In Women, and the first patient, Judith Rochford, was admitted. Now known as the Rotunda Hospital, its doors have never since closed and over 6000 women deliver there each year. The hospital continues to fulfil its two great objectives - to help the poor and needy and to teach its pupils how best that help can be given.

The birth of the hospital was entirely due to the vision and energies of its remarkable founder, then only in his thirty-third year, Bartholomew Mosse. Although lacking substantial personal wealth, he displayed a single minded resolve. He had previously received his papers as a surgeon in 1733 and studied in Holland, France and England. Having become a Licentiate in Midwifery in 1742, the dismay he experienced on seeing the conditions under which women delivered inspired him to undertake his great venture.

His secretary Higgins described how "In the course of his practice, charity often demanded his assistance and he often declared that the misery of the poor women of the city of Dublin at the time of their lying-in would scarcely be conceived by anyone who had not been an eyewitness to their wretched circumstances; their lodgings were generally in cold garrets open to every wind, or in damp cellars subject to flooding from excessive rain; destitute of attendance, medicine, and often of proper food by virtue of which hundreds perished with their little infants."

To raise the income needed, Mosse showed a flamboyant entrepreneurial spirit. To augment the funds he was able to generate from wealthy patrons, he raised money by rather high risk lotteries and brought Europe's leading musicians to play at the concerts he arranged. He was invited to advise those in London who were to follow his lead and to open the British Lying-In Hospital in Brownlow Street, London in 1749 and the following year the City of London Maternity Hospital.

Whilst he might have been expected to spend some time consolidating the prospects of success for his first hospital in George Street, the restless Mosse had greater dreams. Within three years, in 1748, he had acquired the lease on a little over four acres at the top of what is now O'Connell Street, Dublin's main thoroughfare, and engaged the leading architect in Ireland at that time, the German Richard Cassells, to help make his dream become a reality.

By 1757 the new hospital was completed, though Mosse had little time to see the results for in 1759 he died after a short illness in his forty-seventh year. His creation however thrives as living evidence of the fruits that can accrue from caring and concern for others. Within the building, with its rather austere Palladian style, is an architectural gem - the Chapel of exquisite beauty and exuberant decoration, which continues to express Mosse's aspirations as expressed by the Italian stucco artist, Bartholomew Cramillion. Illustrations of three of the figures adorning the alcoves below the ceiling are included later in this book - firstly as a glimpse of the Chapel's inspiring interior and secondly as symbols that we can use when we seek to understand the basis of good childbirth.

From Mosse's endeavours, the first great instance of real caring for women in childbirth, we move forward nearly two hundred years to find the second - the writings of Dr Grantly Dick-Read. His inspiration, his road to Damascus, came from a woman whose labour he was attending at her home in Whitechapel in London. She declined his offer of chloroform, instead looking after herself in her first labour without undue problem. After her delivery, he asked her why she didn't want chloroform and her classic answer was "It didn't hurt. It wasn't meant to, was it?"

This statement formed such a contrast to the torrid painful labours that he usually witnessed. He concluded that fear was the trigger to tension and that tension led to pain. In 1933 he produced his first text 'Natural Childbirth' showing how shedding the element of fear was the first necessary ingredient to a good experience in labour. His views at first encountered extraordinary hos-

Good Childbirth

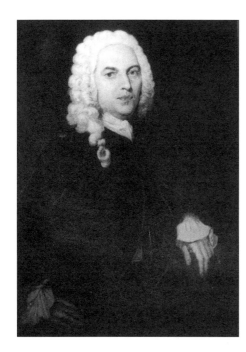

Fig I
Bartholomew Mosse

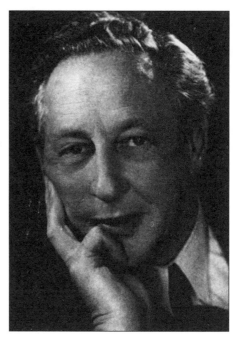

Fig II
Grantly Dick-Read

tility, but then obtained a measure of acceptance and much of the enlightenment that has emerged in the last sixty years is the result of his works.

But today, good labours are still the exception rather than the rule. Still too many expectant women expect their labours to be painful and when their labours arrive, these expectations are realised. There is a simple reason why women continue to have painful labours, even if they have looked at the principles Dick-Read outlined. They may have felt they discarded their fears, but if so they have only done so at a very superficial level. Deep down their fears and anxieties are as firmly embedded as they were before the pregnancy started.

If it was inevitable that every expectant woman was going to have a painful labour, there would be no point in this book. But even on their own initiative a small number of women do manage to have good labours, with a level of discomfort that they find they can absorb and tolerate. In this book, I hope to show you how to join that happy band. When I worked at the Rotunda in 1972, my observations mirrored those of Dick-Read. Since entering general practice nineteen years ago, I have evolved a means of preparation that has allowed many women to help themselves to have a labour that has been a rich and memorable experience. The feedback from these women has produced many of the ideas that are presented in the pages that follow. My hope is that from these pages you will be able to help yourself in such a way that your labour will be everything you would want it to be.

Your pregnancy is like a journey, one of the greatest journeys of your life. To help yourself prepare for the climax of that journey, come on another journey through these pages - a journey of discovery about yourself. Find out which strategies you find help you most in your preparation. Enjoy discovering within yourself abilities which you have always had but only now have learnt to access. Above all, enjoy having the pregnancy and labour you deserve.

Chapter Two

Where have we gone wrong?

It's already puzzled you. You have heard stories of labour from a variety of your friends. To be fair, for some there were factors that meant a mechanically normal labour wasn't on the cards. If it's a first labour and the baby is big meaning big, or if the pelvis is genuinely narrow, or if the baby's head instead of being nicely flexed (chin on chest) is straightened or even extended, then it isn't surprising that they had a lousy time.

But if we put aside those where one of the above possibilities applied and the 'presentation formula' was abnormal, what happens to the rest? This is the baffling part. Look at all your friends who appeared to have everything set fair for a good labour when they have been having their first baby. Bear in mind that everything in this chapter is about women having their first baby, which presents the real challenge to contractions that need to stretch tissues that haven't been stretched before. It means a lot of work for the body but some women do show that it can be done effectively and in a manageable way.

Some, sadly not the majority, have had a good labour. Their contractions even though strong were tolerable to a certain extent - sometimes they needed some help, sometimes they didn't. But the great feature for these women is that they made progress and they 'cracked on'. The contractions might have been good and strong to the point of hurting, but they did their job of dilating and opening up the neck of the womb, so they were worthwhile.

What about the others? They have a tale of woe to tell. And don't they just tell it! The ones who had a good time seem almost bashful about their experiences, but if you had a stinker, the more people you can imprint your rough time upon the better. This may seem a harsh view point, but this imprint does play a part in determining the labour the listener is going to have in her time.

The woman who had a lousy labour had contractions of frightening intensity, that seemed to make her feel as if she was tearing

Good Childbirth

herself to bits. The distressing feature for the woman is that these contractions didn't work. After a few hours of these slammers, the neck of womb had hardly dilated at all. She felt an overwhelming despair. Labour is a vulnerable enough time without going through all that for no gain.

But it doesn't need to be like that. Given an average size pelvis, average size baby presenting by the head which is reasonably flexed, it should be a realisable goal for most women to have the first type of labour I have outlined.

When you come to a pond that's frozen over, you always have to put one foot on the ice to test it. If it feels strong, you go a bit further. Here's where I put a foot onto the ice of the various women's movements who are probably indignant that this book is being written by a man in the first place. In response to that point I can only say that it has been asking to be written since women started having lousy labours with normal presentations and if no woman's got around to it, then I should!

Come with me along this line of reasoning which I feel has a strong thread of truth running through it. Don't get vexed at the comparisons between humans and animals - the comparisons are constructive. Look at what we are designed to do - the fact that some women achieve it proves that it can be achieved. Look at what we so often end up doing - we don't need to end up there and if we did it would give us a rotten experience instead of the good one we deserve.

What have we as humans in common with other animals in the class called mammals? We all have a uterus (womb) in which the fetus grows until ready for delivery. Look down a microscope at the muscle fibres of the womb of a human and another large mammal and you'd be hard put to tell the difference. Study the mechanics of the contractions and they are much the same in any mammal including humans They exert an organised forceful effect on the neck of the womb, opening and dilating it and forming the birth canal ready for delivery.

If you stand on your cat's foot or your dog traps her tail in the door, the animal can and will make a noise reflecting the pain it experiences. If normal labour in animals was intrinsically painful, you can be sure that the animal would make the same noise. It wouldn't feel embarrassed about making the noise and keep silent. It wouldn't worry about what anyone would think if it made the noise. If normal labour hurt that much, the animal would make the 'I am in pain' noise.

But it doesn't. Watch an animal in labour. You can tell something is going on. It is restless and is experiencing its contractions but the message that is coming from the womb, along the nerves and up the spinal cord to the brain is not that of intense severe pain. If it was, the animal would surely make 'the pain noise'.

Some people might say "But we are humans, we are different, labour in humans is bound to be painful." Two facts show that this is not true. Firstly the fact that from the spinal cord down we humans are the same as other mammals and therefore from the base of the brain and the spinal cord down we have at least the potential to have the same experience as other mammals. Secondly the fact that a proportion of first time women do manage to achieve the good labour that they do and that therefore it lies within the compass of attainment of so many more of us humans.

If no woman could have a good labour, I wouldn't be writing this book. If all women with a normal presentation had a good labour, I wouldn't be writing this book. The reason I am writing it is to try to show you what you can achieve if you trust yourself and get both yourself and your thinking into the right frame.

Some parts of your body are very sensitive and have sophisticated nerve endings. With your eyes closed you can tell if you are brushing your finger tip over cotton wool or silk or wood. A painful stimulus to your finger tip such as a splinter of wood going under your nail or a burn is immediately and intensely painful. This is useful as in an instant you would pull your finger away by reflex action.

Other parts of your body have different types of nerve endings. 'Inside' bits generally have less sophisticated nerve endings. That's not to say they can't let you know what's going on. They can and they do. Good contractions that start up near the top of the womb and work down like a wave to open up and dilate the neck of the womb will let you know they are there. Unless they are over strong, there is every prospect of their being manageable with a real prospect of no outside help being required.

Good Childbirth

Lousy contractions that are truly painful and that don't make progress start in the lower part of the womb and spread to the rest of the womb, but they don't exert any useful opening effect on the neck of the womb. The lower part of the womb has more sensitive nerve endings - these are the ones triggering off messages when you have bad dysmenorrhoea or painful periods. Anyone who has had that will confirm that there are real pain fibres in the lower part of the womb! Talk to women who have had good contractions - even when they are strong they are that bit different to the dysmenorrhoea message or the lousy contraction message.

You can take it as a general guide that if your body is working normally, it isn't painful. Of course it isn't as simple as that. Apply any stimulus with a greater and greater force and it will eventually become intolerable to the level of experiencing pain - that doesn't mean the stimulus is in itself painful, just that it has been increased to such a pitch that it becomes painful it has gone above my 'pain threshold'.

Think of someone putting their arms around you and squeezing you with increasing strength. At first it is barely perceptible - you can just feel the arms. A bit more squeeze and depending on whose arms they are, you might describe it as pleasant. More squeeze and it becomes uncomfortable. More squeeze and you find it unpleasant to the point you want it to stop. More squeeze and it genuinely is painful.

Let's apply this model to labour. In a good labour there is nothing to fear about having strong contractions. Ten good strong contractions can make as much progress as forty weak ones. The stronger they are and the longer they last, the more prospect there is of my making progress. There are times when good strong contractions are so strong that they spend so long above my pain threshold that I find them difficult to manage - that's when I ask for and get some help. That's down to common sense.

The message in this book is that so long as you give yourself the good strong co-ordinated contractions that will make progress for you and your baby, you can have a labour that might be hard work, as the word labour suggests, but you will have every prospect of staying on top of these contractions and you can have an experience that will be good to look back at.

How can you 'give yourself' good contractions? Until now you've looked at yourself from the base of the brain, down the spinal cord and along the nerves to the muscle tissue of the womb. To work out how to give yourself good contractions we've got to go the other way into the brain and look at what happens there. This is where all your friends have led themselves astray and where you can sort out your thinking so you will be able to look after yourself, your feelings and your contractions.

Good Childbirth

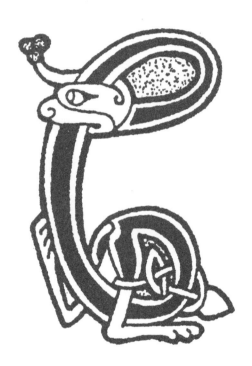

Chapter Three

How we start off on the wrong foot

In the last chapter you have sensed how things should work from the base of the brain down. You've comprehended how from the womb up to the base of the brain you should have every prospect of having a good labour. Where do humans go wrong?

Well, the answer is above the base of the brain. After all it is the brain that distinguishes humans from other animals. Overall this is something to be thankful for. It gives us intelligence, reasoning, affection and emotions far beyond the reach of other animals.

It has allowed us to develop language, the ability to create and construct beyond imagination and to adapt our environment to our needs. At the same time it seems to have created a potential for destruction and cruelty particularly towards other members of our own species that can only generate a sense of despair.

When we look at what it has done for our ability to labour, it really gets interesting. My understanding of why we get a lousy labour is based on supposition and deduction, but let yourself absorb the line of thinking I will set out for you and you'll find yourself saying "OK, I see what he's getting at - it makes sense to me - how can I use these ideas to help myself?".

I believe that there are two main concepts that will allow you to have the labour you deserve - firstly you want to be able to accept the message from good contractions without distorting that message into something worse or different - secondly you want to recondition your innermost thinking so that you actually give yourself a strong likelihood of having good contractions instead of lousy ones. A fairly mind blowing prospect, but until now you haven't known the half of what you can do.

Good Childbirth

Although she is blindfolded, her feet rest upon a sure base and she has the unfailing comfort of the Cross and Bible. The fox, the enemy of the vine, is crushed beneath her foot as she suspends the plummet of righteousness above the coiled serpent. Denied the comfort of sight, she is nevertheless able to put her trust in the protection given unto her.

You can have justifiable faith in yourself and the way you are designed to be able to have a good labour. Your body can and will look after your labour if you have enough confidence in yourself and your body to leave everything to get on with its job in the way it is designed to do. This calls for a lot of trust in yourself but it is one of the mainstays of how to create the setting within yourself to have the kind of labour you deserve.

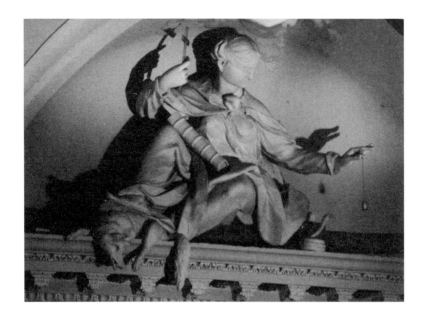

Fig III   FAITH

In the alcove beneath the ceiling of the Chapel of the
Rotunda Hospital Dublin - East Wall

Good Childbirth

CONCEPT ONE: I want to accept my contractions for what they are without distorting them into something they are not.

I hope you can accept that humans and animals are the same from the base of the brain down. Given a favourable 'presentation formula' for labour, the messages coming up my spinal cord should be that I am having good strong contractions that are making progress. If I had a simple brain that would probably be all that would happen. I would perceive I was in labour and get into some shelter and lie down.

But I have a great big brain that can do lots of things. How I perceive things is now much more complicated than just accepting the message that comes up my spinal cord. I have produced this formula to explain what I mean:

$$P = S + E$$

'P' means perception - what I make of what is going on. 'S' is the stimulus - the basic message that has come into my brain, whether up my spinal cord, through my hearing system or through my vision. 'E' is the mixture of experience and emotion that my brain produces as an additional dimension - this mixture modifies the stimulus to produce my perception.

What does this gobbledygook mean? Let's look at an example. You are sitting at home in a brightly lit room, enjoying a light snack watching Coronation Street. Your beloved husband who is wandering through the room behind your seat, soon to go off out to play darts, stands behind you and says the word "Boo". The only stimulus that has come into your brain is the word "Boo" via your ear. You haven't had any visual or tactile stimulus. You hear the word "Boo" and your perception is: "What a twerp!"

Now look at the same stimulus in a different setting, later the same night. Hubbie isn't back from his darts yet and you're not expecting him for some time. You're sitting in darkness now, curled up with a cushion, watching that most frightening of all horror movies 'Dracula meets Frankenstein in the Crypt of Horrors.' It's just coming up to the moment where the lid of the coffin slides back and you dread to even guess what might happen next.

Unbeknownst to you, hubbie has returned early and has come to stand behind you. Barely able to suppress his snigger, he provides the same solitary stimulus to your brain, the word "Boo". And what happens? In just one millisecond, the computer that is your brain takes that stimulus and adds to it all the emotion and experience you possess. You are in a state of anxiety and dread from the film. Your brain knows that hubbie is out and here is an intruder threatening violence and rape and heaven knows what else. Before this even gets anywhere near your consciousness, you find yourself emitting a piercing shriek and leaping out of your seat.

Your perception was the blend of the stimulus and your experience and emotion. Let's apply this to labour. Up my spinal cord comes a message saying "I am now having a good strong contraction." What most women now do is add to that stimulus the host of imprints and influences that they have consciously and subconsciously received in the years before this pregnancy. First we'll look at these imprints and then we'll reframe them into something more useful.

And when you look at these imprints it isn't surprising that the perception of the stimulus is lousy. Think back to every time you have seen any film or television programme of a labouring woman in a dramatic story and what have you seen? She is thrashing around, screaming blue murder as everyone seeks without success to restrain her. With an agonising wail she expels this frightening load and sobs inconsolably. You were only fourteen when you saw this for the first time, but in your subconscious you'll never forget it.

I should point out that I'm not into all this politically correct rubbish. I couldn't care less if a chairman of a meeting is male or female - the word chairman will do for me and I'm not going to alter my use of words just to avoid upsetting some group. For me the thing in the middle of the road will always be a manhole cover and I'm not going to start calling it a person hole cover for anyone. At school my daughters will study history not hertory.

Good Childbirth

Seated in the alcove opposite Faith, she builds on her sister's blindfolded trust. Comforted by that strength, her open eyes are uplifted to the heavens. Her left hand is in a position of supplication as her right rests on the anchor that secures her beliefs.

Given that you allow youself to have faith in yourself and in the way normal labour can and should progress, you may then allow yourself to have hope that the fates will indeed deal you a good hand. There is no sure prospect of this but the way you have prepared yourself after taking on board the ideas in this book gives you the greatest prospect that your labour will turn out to be everything you would hope for.

Good Childbirth

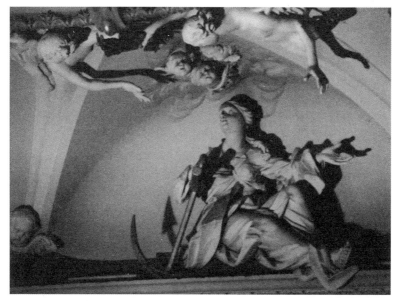

Fig IV   HOPE

In the alcove beneath the ceiling of the Chapel of the
Rotunda Hospital Dublin - West Wall

But it has to be said the vocabulary that we have given labour doesn't help. Labour starts when your 'pains' are regular, how are your 'pains' now, when do you want some 'painkillers', what were your 'pains' like, my 'pains' were terrible and so on. I can understand how this has crept in, but it isn't fair to the first time pregnant woman who should be starting with a clean sheet. I can understand another woman who had a lousy labour in the past using such words - they reflect the unfortunate experience she had - but by using and promoting this kind of vocabulary she isn't being fair to the first timer who has never had labour contractions. By the use of such a vocabulary, we are introducing the untrue premise that contractions have to be painful, but of course we know from the experience of those women who labour well that this does not have to be so.

From being a child I remember what a pain is - when I had that ear infection, that great big boil on my neck, when I caught my finger in a door. Now you tell me I am going to have pains in labour, so I start subconsciously recalling all the 'pains' I have ever had. How bad are these contractions going to be? I can't stand them and they haven't even started yet. It would be really helpful if women who had a lousy time stopped telling anyone at all about their experience and if all those concerned with looking after expectant women - doctors, midwives, health visitors and anyone else - took a long hard look at the vocabulary they use and the imprint it must make. Look at the positive gain that comes from calling contractions what they are - contractions - and not using a word like 'pain' that brings with it such a lot of preconditioning.

It isn't surprising that every first timer takes deeply on board the imprint from her own mother. Tell me mum, what it was like when you had me? If the mother had a lousy time and gives a lurid account, you can bet the daughter is halfway to a lousy time herself. Even if the mother clamps her lips, her daughter will pick up an awareness that a grotty event happened to her mother then and that the same grotty event now lies ahead for her. Furthermore all the torrid tales her friends have told her must push her thinking into the expectation that she is going to have a lousy time as well.

Many women have confided in me one underrated factor that generates fear - the perception of their own internal configuration.

Good Childbirth

From early teens, perhaps having the occasional struggle with tampons, they have had an idea of the dimensions and space 'inside.' But hold on a minute - look at the size of this baby and in particular its head. How on earth can that get through - there is just no way. It is a great act of faith for the woman (and for the doctors and midwives!) to take on board the reality that all her own tissues can and will move out of the way to form a huge birth canal that will give enough space for the baby to slide easily and safely through. But it is true - all you have to do is believe in yourself and let it happen on its own.

It's a shame that labour is such an unknown thing - I can't work out in advance what it's going to be like - I can't really rehearse or practice - then on the day suddenly bang, here it is and off we go with no going back. This creates its own fear and dread. It takes a lot of faith in the design of things and in your own ability to cope to trust yourself and your body in labour.

One of my big fears is of losing control. I don't want to be helpless, unable to cope, to let myself down, to be a failure. Yet by allowing these thoughts to get embedded, I am almost encouraging these developments to happen. Of course there is no real reason why any of them should happen and if I trust myself there is every reason to expect that I can remain in charge of myself and my feelings and reactions.

Here's an example of the unhelpful ways women find their thoughts misleading them. "That was such an awful painful contraction that I felt I was going to burst." If it was a real slammer of a contraction, it happened anyway. Why not say to yourself: "That was a really strong contraction, so strong it made me feel like bursting. But of course I can't burst - instead it must have been such a strong one that it must really have done a lot of good in helping me make progress." Easier said than done, but it is a better way of coping with the real slammers if that is what you get.

Many women feel fearful about the unknown issue - How long is this labour going to take? It's worth bearing in mind that there's a lot of 'preparing the way' that has to be done in the first stage. Tissues that haven't before been stretched before have to be stretched now to allow them to move out of the way. These days we seem to have lost sight of the simple truth that this can take time. For a woman having her first labour, the first stage can often take ten or twelve hours, even when it is progressing nicely under its own steam.

How long is this labour going to take? Well of course in real terms it doesn't really matter how long it takes, because as long as I am coping with the contractions and I am in charge of myself, time doesn't really matter. I can day dream, looking back at happy memories or looking ahead to when I see my baby for the first time. And as I day dream, time just seems to pass. Of course if I'm screaming blue murder then every second seems like eternity and I want to know when will it ever end. In lousy labours time matters a lot, but in good labours it doesn't really seem to matter at all.

When I'm anxious everything hurts. Look at the kid raising the roof when Jimmy kicked him. He's frightened at the shock to his system and he's hurt. His mother cuddles him and talks to him, the crying suddenly stops and his troubled face clears, a little choked up laugh blurting out as he chooses a strawberry ice cream and he wipes away the now unnecessary tear. If I'm anxious and frightened going into labour, my contractions will hurt like mad. If I'm at peace within, the same contractions come and go and I float along with them. If I'm tired when I go into labour, my contractions will feel worse than they would do if I arrive well rested and looking forward to one of the greatest days of my life.

These are just some of the imprints that were set in the subconscious even before you started your pregnancy, never mind before you came to your labour. Any or all of these factors have the potential to convert the simple message coming up your spinal cord - "I am having good strong contractions" - into a terrifying "I am having dreadful pains that are killing me". However this conversion is neither necessary nor helpful and in later chapters you can learn how to free yourself of this converting tendency and restore yourself to the straightforward direct uncomplicated person you really are.

You need to comprehend that it is almost certain that by the time you come to be pregnant, you will have had these imprints embedded in your subconscious, even though your conscious awareness might suggest to you that you have not. This book will show you how to break free from this state of affairs and give yourself the labour you deserve. To help you comprehend what changes you need to make within yourself, I want to introduce a new expression to use when we are talking about all the imprints and expectations that you have. We could use an expression that already exists like 'frame of mind', but if we use a pre-existing expression we will adopt the implications it already carries. I prefer to use a new fresh expression to cover the overall contents of your embedded thoughts. This expression is your 'cerebral pitch'.

Your 'cerebral pitch' will be the end result of all your thoughts, conscious and subconscious, and will determine how you approach your labour and how you cope with your contractions. But it is even more important than that. As we will see in the rest of this chapter and in the next, your cerebral pitch can actually determine what kind of labour you get. It's beginning to get exciting. Let's read on.

CONCEPT TWO - If you have an unfavourable cerebral pitch, you will have a lousy labour. If you unlearn the unfavourable cerebral pitch and learn a favourable cerebral pitch, you then have a great prospect of having a good labour.

The first step is to understand how we learn many things. The sequence is firstly conscious learning which is then followed by subconscious learning. Now the problem is that once we have completed the process of subconscious learning, we cannot easily undertake subconscious unlearning from the conscious state. We need to access our subconscious so that we can undergo subconscious unlearning followed by relearning and this is the key process we must seek to achieve.

To see what I mean, cast your mind back to how you learnt to drive your car. First you underwent conscious learning. You learnt how to listen to the noise the engine was making as you pressed the accelerator down a bit more, then you eased your foot off the clutch and the car shuddered forwards as you squeezed the death out of the steering wheel. As time passed you found that you needed to pay less and less attention to the engine noise and before long it seemed second nature. You had by now undergone subconscious learning in this and all the other aspects of driving.

Good Childbirth

Charity means caring and love. Here the seated figure suckles her newborn as her other children play about her. Her serenity and joy are evident as she now gives the babe a continuation of the nourishment she gave before birth. Angels stretch down their hands in support and cherubs rejoice in the giving of new life.

You can look forward to giving new life, to succouring the newborn and to experiencing a new plane, indeed a new rich depth, in your life. It is towards this fulfilment that your pregnancy is leading and your labour is to be the means of opening that door. Your faith in yourself and your hope based on that faith set the scene on what has a real prospect of being one of the greatest days in your life.

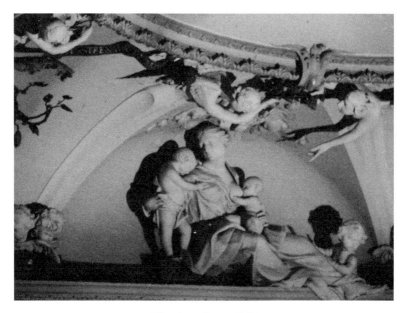

Fig V   CHARITY

In the alcove beneath the ceiling of the Chapel of the
Rotunda Hospital Dublin - South Wall

Good Childbirth

What is your driving like now? You don't listen to the engine noise at all, you change gear while you are talking to your passenger. You go round a corner safely and in control and yet if I asked you a few yards further on whether you were in second or third gear you wouldn't know. Your subconscious learning is complete and your subconscious looks after you safely. Sometimes on the motorway you find you have driven some way without being aware whether or not you have passed junction 6 - yet you were safe at all times.

My contention is that every expectant woman has been exposed to all the unfavourable imprints we have talked about earlier this chapter - these have been passed from the conscious to the subconscious and are now embedded as subconscious learning. This process seems to 'alter the thermostat' and instead of having a good labour with good effective contractions, she is now doomed to having lousy painful contractions that hurt like mad and don't make progress.

To have the good labour you deserve, you have to unlearn at a subconscious level all these imprints, shed them and replace them with a good set of favourable helpful imprints that have one great thing in their favour - they are all true.

There are lots of different ideas about how our minds work. I have to say I don't know if any of them are valid or not, but that doesn't matter to me and I suggest it doesn't need to matter to you. To begin to comprehend how you can help yourself, you can draw on some of these ideas in a way that is useful to you, but there is no need to get too bogged down. Life is too short.

One idea is based on the way the two different halves of our brains behave. The concept is that if you are right handed, the left side of your brain not only tells your right side to move but also is the half of the brain that is responsible for reasoning, analysing and logical thought. The right hand half of the brain by contrast is then the side responsible for imagination, for creative thought, for flair.

Going a little further, the conscious mind can be viewed as being in the left brain and the subconscious in the right. The problem for our purposes is we cannot readily get some new thoughts into the right brain. The usual sequence is that a new thought goes into the left half of the brain first, then may or may not be passed through onto the right. But the left acts like a filter or blocker and the good new thoughts have little chance of getting through to the right brain where they are needed.

As a consequence, all the good work done at antenatal relaxation classes and the like is prevented from getting to where it is needed in the subconscious, embedded in the right brain. All the unfavourable thoughts embedded in the subconscious have got to be uprooted and cast out first. In general terms we don't usually have access to our subconscious and we find we can't do this. In the next few chapters we are going to learn how to achieve subconscious unlearning, and then we will really start getting somewhere.

For our purposes it doesn't matter if all this left-right stuff is true or a load of cobblers. As long as it gives you a mechanism that makes sense to you about how your mind works and what you need to do to get your own subconscious unlearning and relearning under way, that is all that matters.

Good Childbirth

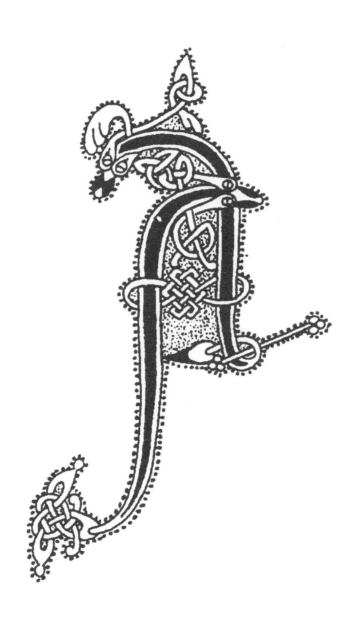

Chapter Four

A good labour or a lousy labour - What's the difference?

It all hinges on whether your contractions are co-ordinated or not. For this chapter I'm afraid it's thinking caps on so you can understand what is meant by:

'UNCO-ORDINATED UTERINE ACTION'

Yes, I know it's a horrible mouthful, but bear with me. Once you've grasped it, you'll see that it is the best term for a phenomenon that lies at the heart of determining whether you have a good labour or a lousy labour.

From the starting point of having all the various elements ready - an average size baby, presenting by the head, the head reasonably flexed and a pelvis of adequate proportions - then the crucial thing that you need to add is a series of good strong co-ordinated contractions and then labour can and will progress.

Once you have absorbed the key thoughts of this book, this is what you can allow to happen in your labour. Trusting your contractions to do their job, on their own, by themselves, as they are so beautifully designed to do, your labour can progress effectively without your experiencing more discomfort than you can absorb. This can be described as a labour with co-ordinated uterine action.

To understand what you are aiming for in your labour, look at the other side of the coin - the labour that is experienced by all too many, when the whole event is dominated by unco-ordinated uterine action. Even with all things set fair, the sequence is all too common. You will already have heard it from your friends. I always feel it is a shame because so often it didn't really need to happen.

As we work together throughout this book, it is important that we avoid the pitfall of 'analysis and paralysis' and most of the time I'm avoiding getting bogged down in too much in the way of explanations. But here we aren't analysing - instead we are comprehending. It is important for you to have a clear grasp of the two different types of labour I am describing and know which one is the one for you.

Let's be clear what labour should mean. It isn't only having regular strong contractions. If you are labouring, you have also got to be making progress. Labour is the package of regular strong contractions that bring the baby's head down through the pelvis and stretch up the cervix to form the birth canal. If you ain't making progress you ain't labouring - you're just having contractions that aren't getting you anywhere,

You want a clear idea of the kind of contractions and the kind of labour you want. To be useful your contractions must be co-ordinated, in the same way that the eight members of a tug of war team must be. They have to all pull together at the same time in an organised purposeful way.

Co-ordinated contractions start near the upper part of the womb and spread like a wave down towards the lower part. At the same time the part of the womb just above the cervix (the 'lower segment') almost seems to relax. The result is that the lower segment is stretched and thinned out and the pull of the good co-ordinated contraction thins out the cervix and then dilates it up. Clever stuff - organised, powerful and effective.

What about the other type of contractions - they are unco-ordinated and are very different. When this is the type of contractions a woman is getting, she can be said to be having unco-ordinated uterine action. The wave of contractions seem to start from the lower part of the womb - the fancy term used is a loss of polarity. There is a high rise of pressure in the inside of the womb and even in between contractions the resting pressure is high. But there is no relaxation of the lower segment. There is no stretching and dilating force applied to the lower segment and cervix. It is a lousy contraction and makes for a lousy labour - and it just doesn't work.

In such a case, the labour is likely to be genuinely painful. The woman isn't making it up - it hurts like hell. The contractions seem to work up to an agonising peak and her back joins in. From the starting point of two centimetres or whatever dilated, after several hours of these screamers, it seems incredible that she is still only two centimetres dilated.

In the days before epidurals, this nightmare went on for many hours with pethidine at frequent intervals but without much effect. Eventually either the baby got distressed at four centimetres dilatation and was delivered by Caesarean section or the woman got to full dilatation and a rather tired and perhaps distressed baby was delivered by forceps.

Nowadays the scenario has moved on, but still is less than satisfactory. These days the woman has an epidural after the second examination has shown little progress despite these slamming ineffective contractions. Now we are into high tech and although life might be rendered bearable, do bear in mind that high tech labours are an entirely different ball game.

At this stage, if the woman is lucky, the removal of her awareness of her contractions can remove the actual trigger to unco-ordinated action. The contractions might then become co-ordinated and effective and her labour becomes the progressive force it is meant to be. More often however the labour plods along, still with unco-ordinated uterine action, albeit with a woman no longer scraping the paint off the walls, and ends with a forceps or vacuum delivery.

I should mention that there is one pain in the neck situation that can make unco-ordinated uterine action rather more likely to arise (but not inevitable!), and that is when the back of the baby's head (the 'occiput') is towards the back of the woman's pelvis when labour starts. The fancy name for this is occipito-posterior or 'OP' and it can sometimes be a bit of a bitch.

It is more common than most people realise for the baby to start off in this position. If that happens to you, what you've got to do is slacken yourself off and let time pass. As long as you go with your labour, you give your contractions a chance of staying co-ordinated, even while the occiput is towards the back You might find that a lot of what you feel is in the back and it has to be said it's not much fun. Pethidine seems to be quite useless for this, but good rubbing seems to help as much as anything. In time your co-ordinated uterine action helps the occiput move round towards the front as labour progresses and you may sense that your contractions have come round to the front and that things are getting going. The occiput then delivers under the bone at the front of your pelvis (the 'pubis'). There are times when the baby finds it easier to have the occiput go further round the back and the face of the baby comes through under the pubis - the 'face-to-pubes' delivery - which can be more of a heave ho for the woman but can still be manageable.

Later in this chapter you can read an account of an occipito-posterior labour as it should be at its most reasonable and an unco-ordinated labour as it all too often is.

Before we do that let's run through the two different types of labour again. It is so crucial that you comprehend the difference. Allow yourself to understand in a deep down way the difference between the two. Put them on a table in front of you like a choice of dessert at a swanky restaurant. Decide which one you want and feel good as you reach out and grab it.

Co-ordinated uterine action (CUA) means what it says. All the muscle fibres of the main part of the uterus start tightening up in an effective co-ordinated way, like a tug-of-war team. Their sustained contraction is delivered down onto the lower part ('lower segment') of the uterus and the neck of womb ('cervix'). Each long strong contraction pulls up the lower segment thinning it out (a process called 'effacing'). The opening of the cervix is drawn more and more open - the process of dilatation - so that from the one or two centimetres starting point as an opening, it is progressively dilated all the way up to ten centimetres which is full dilatation.

In co-ordinated uterine action, the end of a contraction is not followed by elastic recoil to where things were before it started. Instead there is, after the contraction, only partial relaxation of the length of the muscle fibres. The fancy name for this is retraction. It's a bit like men pulling up an anchor on the old sailing ships. They give a strong co-ordinated pull, all working together and lift the anchor a few feet. But instead of letting it fall back onto the sea bed, they have at the height of the pull passed the rope back to keep the anchor lifted. When the next pull comes, they raise the anchor another few feet and again consolidate the newly gained position.

This is what you want to do - give your cervix a good drawing pull with each contraction to open it a bit more and then keep your gain so you don't have to do it all again. Remember your definition of labour - a series of good, strong, co-ordinated contractions that lead to the progressive dilatation of the cervix and formation of the birth canal. This is what you need and this is what you can achieve if you just trust your contractions and let them do their job on their own by themselves.

Unco-ordinated uterine action (UUA) provides a sharp contrast with the above. I'm not talking about the concept that obstetricians mean when they use the term inco-ordinate uterine action - they are talking about the dramatic end stage of what I am looking at. What I am dealing with are the all too common contractions that start in the lower part of the womb and spread upwards. Looked at on the monitor they look quite impressive, with big pressure waves. However they don't seem to be sustained like the waves in co-ordinated uterine action. But just look at how high they went. And wow, did they hurt. So they must be really effective.

But this is the sad bit. Unco-ordinated uterine action not only is painful but it's also useless. Contraction after contraction spends ages above my pain threshold and they are agony. The drawback is they don't make any progress. My cervix stays stubbornly unchanged or makes pitifully slow progress. Any advance I might make at the peak of a contraction is lost because I don't achieve any retraction. To put it mildly it is a dead loss.

Sometimes there is a reason for UUA. If a labour starts as occipito-posterior, UUA seems to occur more readily and only when the baby rotates does the process switch to CUA. My feeling is that the biggest trigger to UUA is the woman's 'cerebral pitch' we have talked about - the outcome of all the imprints she has loaded in that were discussed in Chapter Three. Get rid of those and you have a good prospect of CUA - leave them in and UUA is on the cards. This is why acupuncture and TENS and the like which can raise the levels of the body's own pain killers called endorphins can only help in a proportion of cases - those cases where the woman's cerebral pitch is favourable - but can do little when the woman's pitch is still cluttered with unhelpful and untrue imprints.

In Figs VI and VII you can see the two different shapes to the contractions of CUA and UUA. The CUA one lasts for longer and

GOOD CHILDBIRTH

A diagrammatic representation of just what a good contraction is all about. It slowly builds up to its peak and having exerted a powerful drawing and stretching effect on the lower part of the womb and cervix, it subsides to pause before the next strong effective contraction follows. At its very peak it does spend some time a little way above the horizontal line, which indicates the pitch above which a stimulus of increasing strength can be perceived as painful. But because it is only that modest bit above the line and because I understand that a contraction this good and this strong is doing so much good and getting me there quicker than contractions that aren't as strong, I find that I can put up with that perception of pain at the peak. This is the kind of contraction that is a feature of good strong progressive labour - in other words normal labour that is manageable and that gets me ready for delivery.

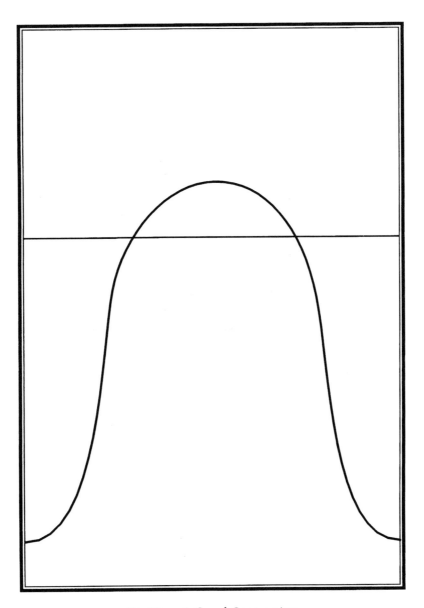

Fig VI   A Good Contraction

Good Childbirth

A diagrammatic representation of the kind of contractions that are all too common and that give the woman a lousy labour. On the monitor they look dramatic and they hurt like hell. They go miles above the threshold over which a stimulus becomes painful. Even in between contractions they don't go back to a resting state. They hurtle up to an agonising peak at the height of each contraction. But they don't work. Hour after hour passes and my cervix is hardly dilating at all. What use are they? The answer is not a lot and it is by the preparation you learn in this book that you reduce the chances of your getting these useless contractions and increase your chance of getting the good ones like the one in Fig VI. So now have your last look ever at this page, satisfy yourself these are not for you and go back to Fig VI and take on board the shape of the contractions you need.

Good Childbirth

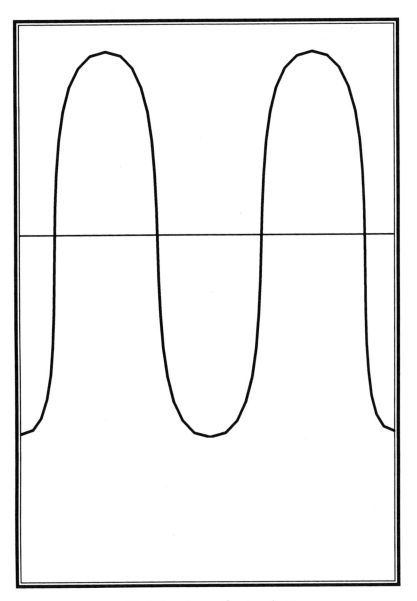

Fig VII   Lousy Contractions

does more good, but is only a bit over your pain threshold. The UUA is way over anyone's pain threshold, however much the body's endorphins have pushed the threshold up. It doesn't last long in a useful way and as far as progress goes is a waste of time. Earlier on we talked about the need for a certain amount of repetition but I think that this chapter has had more than enough. Let's look at what happens in practice.

TONI'S TALE

I was four days over the date I had been given when I went to the antenatal clinic at the hospital. Because my blood pressure was slightly raised they kept me in for induction that evening. I was pleased that I was going to get going at last, but they said the Prostin gel might have to be repeated the next morning and perhaps the afternoon after that. It all sounded a bit drawn out.

When they examined me at 4.30 pm they said I wouldn't need the gel after all, as I was starting off on my own and that made me feel a lot easier. During the evening, after Gavin had gone home, I had spells of backache every ten minutes or so but rubbing my back helped a lot and there wasn't much to feel round the front. Listening to the tape of waves on the seashore helped keep me on an even keel.

My GP bobbed in at 11 pm to see how I was getting on. I felt I was doing well especially when I saw a young girl in the bed opposite. She was screaming the place down and I was relieved when they took her down for an epidural. What lay ahead for me?

By midnight I was still only two centimetres but I couldn't get to sleep. The mixture of backache and excitement meant sleep was miles away. By 1 am the contractions were getting stronger. There was a girl in the bed alongside me who was having her fourth child but she was all over the place. She kept grabbing the sheets with clenched fists and throwing her legs out straight. Even though she was only just getting going she wanted the 'gas and air'. I thought it was meant to be easier when you were having your fourth.

Good Childbirth

At 1.20 am, they moved me down to the delivery suite and Gavin came back to the hospital. I enjoyed sitting in a rocking chair, concentrating on my breathing and going away into my 'happy memories'. The midwives put the monitor on to keep an eye on my progress and encouraged me when they told me how well I was coping with my contractions. My waters broke at 2 am and I was moved onto the delivery bed. The contractions came round to the front now and were pretty strong. The 'gas and air' helped me through a lot at this stage.

When it got to 3 am and I was examined they told me I was only 3-4 cms. I knew I had all options available and had an injection of pethidine but I have to say it didn't give me much relief from the contractions though Gavin said it made me sound drunk. I still had to work hard and concentrate on my breathing. I didn't really like not being aware of what was going on.

At 4 am they examined me again because the baby's heart was slowing down and I knew I was only making slow progress when they told me I was 5 cms. Then the contractions eased off and I began to think I was going off the boil. They sent for the doctor and I felt really good when he examined me at 4.30 am and told me I was 9 centimetres now - I knew I had suddenly made lots of progress and was nearly there.

By ten past five I was fully dilated and by 5.45 am, when the midwife had left the room, I just knew it was time to push - it was an overwhelming urge. No-one could have stopped me! Gavin was worried about the baby's heart rate and the midwife was talking about forceps if I didn't deliver soon, but I knew I could get there with a few more pushes.

They asked me if I wanted to feel his head when it was out but I didn't want to - I just wanted to keep pushing. I felt a bit embarrassed at my 'noise' but they told me I had done really well and not to bother, which made me feel better.

Good Childbirth

The midwives were really helpful which was very important to me and it was great to have Gavin encouraging me all the way.

What about the girl in the next bed at 1 am having her fourth baby? She still hadn't delivered by 7 am.

* * * * * * * * *

I'm not daft enough to pretend that labour is all roses. It's dangerous enough to be writing this book as a non-female who hasn't been in labour. All I will say is that throughout this book what I am presenting is simply the truth upon truth that all the women in the world who have laboured effectively will confirm. Think of the word 'labour' and you think of work, which is what you are ready for. If your neck of womb hasn't been stretched before, it's going to take a lot of work to stretch it. It's going to take a lot of work to guide the baby's head through your pelvis. Up here in the North of England, we're not afraid of work, but for heaven's sake give me good contractions that will do their job.

Just read through Toni's tale again. I think it is a delightful description of an occipito-posterior labour. During the early part, the baby's occiput is round to the back of Toni's pelvis - lots of backache and not much progress. But by 'hanging loose' it stays manageable and it's a matter of waiting for the head to rotate. That happened a little after 4 am - the contractions came round to the front and things really started getting somewhere with rapid dilatation of the cervix and the head coming down - in other words good labour.

As far as I'm concerned, the women I've worked with have a completely free hand. When it comes to the big day, they can do what they want in labour and they know this. In some of the accounts you will see how they come up with their own strategies. So quite a few have a dose of pethidine when they are getting to the flogged stage, but nearly all report that it was pretty useless as regards doing much good. What is good is the gas and air. Not only does it take the edge off the contractions but it still leaves me in control. I can take the mask off my face whenever I want and after a few deep breaths I'm back to wherever I was before.

In Toni's tale we can sense the support from the midwives - that they are really with her and providing caring and capable supervision. They know where she's up to and make sure she knows as well. And can't you tell how it helps?

What about the women with unco-ordinated uterine actions? They were in the beds opposite and alongside Toni, getting nowhere and having a lousy time that they didn't need to have.

Good Childbirth

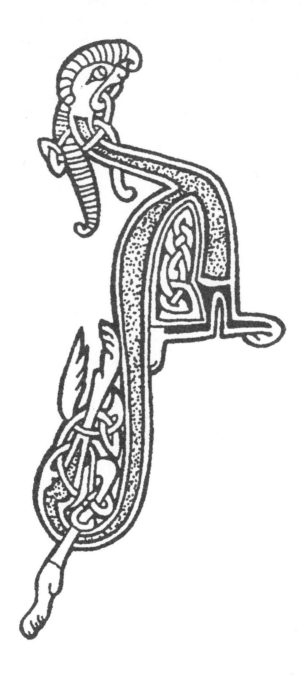

Chapter Five

How do I get the labour I want?

In the last chapter you've learnt the difference between a good labour and a lousy labour. You've learnt how which kind of labour you get is to a large extent determined by your cerebral pitch. You've come to understand how your cerebral pitch is the end result of a process of conscious learning followed by subconscious learning. You sense how in our society and culture nearly everyone gets to adult life with an unfavourable cerebral pitch. They have seen the film and television representation of labour as a terrifying painful event, they have listened to their friends, their mothers have, perhaps inadvertently, transmitted an imprint that labour is awful - so it's not surprising that the odds are stacked against a good labour.

What you seek to do is to cleanse your cerebral pitch, to replace all the unfavourable and untrue imprints with useful, helpful and true anchoring points that will set up the prospects of a good labour when the big day comes. This is more difficult to achieve than you might at first think, but it can be done. To understand why it is difficult, think back to your lessons on computers. The mind is in so many ways like a computer that it's a good analogy. You remember that little tab you slid across to 'write-protect' your discs. When you did that, the information could be read and used, but you couldn't alter it unless you slid the tab back again. The subconscious is a bit like that, and once you've completed subconscious learning it becomes 'write protected'. Subconscious unlearning can be done, but first you've got to access your subconscious and slide back that tab.

It is because subconscious unlearning is a bit of a knack that ordinary efforts to prepare the way for labour are only patchily effective. A straightforward discussion on how labour could be gets nowhere because all the old imprints are left undisturbed. Most of the material presented in the relaxation classes floats through the awareness but nothing has changed deep down.

Good Childbirth

The Americans have a happy ability to take something that is simple and make it complicated. They provide great examples of the 'Analysis and Paralysis' phenomenon which I have mentioned here and there. One of my areas of interest is golf and it is always a source of amazement to me to see an American who has had the benefits of far too many lessons stand practically immobile squeezing the lifeblood out of the club while he recalls his latest tip. Contrast this with the innocence of youth who instinctively grip the club soundly, turn their back on the ball and then sweep it away. I had the good fortune to be guided by a golf teacher who taught through feel and imagination and allowed me to sense the shape of the swing in an 'inside' way. This allowed me to erase and unlearn the faulty building blocks I had previously passed into my subconscious learning and learn anew.

The Americans have gone along the same path with labour. No longer is there a husband. Instead he is now the labour coach ready to instruct the labouring woman as to which of seven types of breathing she is to do at each stage. Each step along the way is analysed and categorised. Depart from the prescribed route and doom will befall you. Several large organisations in this country instill the same formula here with all its inbuilt intensity. Husband and wife emerge exhausted but exultant from each class convinced that they are going to crack it and labour is going to be just fine. Would that it were so.

Instead the outcome is predictable. They have not only failed to complete the subconscious unlearning that we know is needed, but to make things worse have added in the left brain analytical approach. The result is almost predictable to the last detail. Despite a pelvis that could accommodate a ten pound baby without difficulty, the woman 'labours' for seventeen hours by which stage she has reached only four centimetres. Not only is she getting tired but the baby, whose oxygen levels are less than normal during the unco-ordinated labour that has been produced, becomes distressed and a Caesarean section saves the day.

The analytical left brain is all very well for other things in life but when it comes towards preparing for labour we should be talking right brain thinking and subconscious thinking all the way. To access your subconscious learning you seek to access your right brain. In the waking state this is usually blocked by the left brain which acts like a bouncer at a night club. Left brain decides what goes past it and what doesn't. All too often this means that all the good thoughts that right brain needs get dismantled and dispersed by left brain and poor old right brain never gets a sniff of them.

For conditions other than childbirth, the practical way of bypassing left brain and instead working directly with right brain is by medical hypnotherapy. For a variety of conditions from migraine to eczema, medical hypnotherapy has on an individual case basis made many patients' lives bearable once more where mainline medicine has come to an impasse. In the case of childbirth the results are even more emphatic and over the last half century a variety of works have shown how useful it can be. What we should first do is comprehend how hypnotherapy helps in preparation for childbirth and then work out how you are going to help yourself get the labour you deserve without the need for any formal hypnotherapy at all!

BLACK ARTS AND THE STAGE JOHNNIES

Over the next few pages we can look at what hypnotherapy is and what it isn't. You can pick out what elements you want to draw from hypnotherapy that are going to give you the means to achieve the subconscious unlearning that will be the first stage of clearing your mind of all the unfavourable imprints that you want to shed.

Whenever I am providing hypnotherapy for an expectant woman, one thing that really irritates me is that I have to spend a substantial amount of time helping her shed the unfavourable imprints she has about hypnosis in its various aspects. It is an unfortunate truth that nearly everyone has funny ideas about hypnosis and hypnotherapy. Few people seem to realise that the hypnotic state is a normal state of mind that each one of us spends some time in every day.

An example will show you what I mean. Imagine that you have gone to bed early and hubbie is going out to play darts. He comes in to the bedroom and strolls over to the dressing table to collect his keys. You are settled down and not far from slumber, and although you sense that he is there, you decide not to disturb yourself. He looks over and assumes you are asleep, though you know you aren't. But consider two other situations. Firstly, if Bill had rung earlier and asked you to tell John to ring him, you would open your eyes and say "Bill wants you to ring him." John would say "I'll do that - I thought you were asleep." Secondly, if you know John had already gone out, you would sense that there was something wrong and immediately open your eyes ready to challenge any intruder - only to find that John had come back in for his keys!

That's all the hypnotic state really is - not ordinary wakefulness and not asleep - and in itself it's no big deal. What it does however give you is a chance to access your subconscious and introduce the improvements you want to effect there. What you learn to do through proper hypnotherapy is to learn to access your subconscious when you need to for the purposes you want to achieve. Indeed achievement is a key word. Think of the weight lifter coming on to stage to lift great weights. The process he undertakes is based on hypnotic training. When he looks out in front of him, he's not looking for Aunty Gladys in the second row. He's clearing his mind of distractions, of fear of failure, of trying to analyse how to lift this bar. Instead he's visualising the bar rocketing upwards, he's allowing a few weights to fall off each end, he's looking for a surge of his fullest powers. In other words his thinking is completely right brain. The result is that he achieves his full potential. Look at a variety of top sportsmen and sportswomen and you will see echoes of what we have been talking about.

What about the other side of the coin? My instincts tell me that the reason our various national teams fail when they should succeed is largely because they have allowed their thinking to be run from their dominant analytical left brain. They read the papers in the days running up to the event and start brooding and analysing - under achievement is the result. The other team go out and trust in their own ability and play from the creative imaginative right brain and produce stunning results. That's what you want to do in labour. Achieving your own full potential is all you need to look after yourself on the big day.

There appear to be two main sources of the reluctance people have to embark on hypnotherapy - firstly the dramatic representations in fiction, plays and films and secondly those dreadful stage shows. Neither has any substance or relevance but both create impressions that need to be dispelled.

Hypnosis has acquired a false image of one person's mind being controlled by another. The impression is given of the swinging watch, the helpless drift into unconsciousness, the manipulation of the mind of one person by another and a loss of control of oneself - the complete opposite of what actually occurs. What hypnotherapy for childbirth aims for and achieves is providing the expectant woman with more control of herself, her feelings and her reactions. She learns to shed unfavourable imprints that are neither true nor helpful. She learns how to trust her own resources and powers. She learns how to look after herself and to remain in charge of herself and her feelings. And don't forget this - although people will be with you when you are in labour, you need all the ability to manage yourself that you can get. A rotten labour can be a very lonely time.

The really major block to a wider uptake of hypnotherapy is the appalling impression given by the stage and television shows. They create a sense that hypnosis will make a fool out of you, that you are likely to do foolish things and that you are being manipulated. But of course you are not, because you don't take part. What actually does happen is quite different. Imagine that you and I went to one of these shows. I won't call the person running the show a hypnotist, though he may be making use of hypnotic phenomena - let's call him the 'artist'.

Volunteers are called for and there is an avalanche of people rushing onto the stage. It is quite noticeable how most are in their late teens. The secret is that by leaving their seats, all those on the stage have as good as put their names to a consent document. That document says: "Although I haven't been to one of these shows before, I know that you want some people to make a fool of, so everyone will laugh. I want to be one of those people. I want people to laugh at me. I give my consent for you to involve me in this activity."

The next stage is that the 'artist' selects by susceptibility tests those consenting volunteers who have a high capacity for hypnotic activity - in late teenagers these will be quite plentiful - and of course by implication those who have gone onto the stage will be exhibitionists. Now you have all the ingredients for the tasteless shows that blight the general public's perception.

But what if things were different? What if he sent all those who rushed up on the stage back to their seats and tried to work with me, you and all the other people who stayed glued in their seats? Quite simply, he would have no show. By staying in our seats, we made the following statement: "I know something of what you plan, and I don't want to be part of it. I am prepared to laugh at those who will take part but I withhold my consent from my taking any part."

A patient of mine, now elderly, rushed up onto the stage at such a show just after the last war, because he was interested in seeing if he could make part of himself numb - a part of the act he had heard about. He complied with the suggestions given and was delighted to sense how he had so numbed his arm that a needle could be passed through his skin without discomfort. The 'artist' then suggested he kiss the girl next to him. John said "Get lost - I only came to see if I could do the needle bit" and walked off the stage.

Given high capacity consenting young exhibitionists, the events in these shoddy shows are not particularly impressive. They have to my mind as little relevance to the proper use of hypnotherapy as a mode of useful and safe treatment as does a pornographic movie has to the intimate and special moment that leads up to a baby being conceived. You may perceive that I view these stage johnnies as less than the dust beneath the wheels of my chariot.

I am reluctant to waste any more time and space on them and I hope you can shed from your thinking any element of their activities. Let's get back to what really matters.

SO HOW DO I GET THE LABOUR I WANT?

You will remember that I said earlier this chapter that you were going to get the labour you deserve without any actual hypnotherapy and so you shall. You will achieve this by using the scaffolding and principles of hypnotherapy without needing any formal hypnotherapy at all. For this, you and I have to thank a remarkable Canadian doctor called Marlene Hunter. I met her at an Advanced Hypnotherapy course many years ago when she first put me onto a simple truth - if you are pregnant you are in some ways in a hypnotic state all the time throughout your pregnancy and all you have to do is access it.

Think of the hypnotic state as a state of altered awareness - so is pregnancy. In your normal state of awareness you would hardly feel good about having some other being growing inside you. Be aware how you do feel 'different', whether it be more tender, more feeling or something else. Watch a film and sense how you feel the emotions generated within yourself so much more deeply and intensely. The glow of serenity and of achievement are special to pregnancy and some people feel they are gliding through the months. Sense the altered perception of your body - you watch it change and in a way you might feel like a spectator to yourself.

Let the enjoyment of how different you feel be something private and special that you keep to yourself. It's nothing to do with anyone else and anyway it's not easy to put into words. Shona, living in Edinburgh, has managed to put down onto paper a glimpse of how she feels and reading what she has shared with us may help you to access your own inside feelings.

SHONA'S SECRET.

You asked me to put down on paper how I feel about being an expectant mother. Well, from day one my main feeling has been that I have a secret and that it belongs only to me. I know that in time there is going to be another life and that life is always going to belong partly to me. It's as if that little body and my heart hold a secret that will never be spoken about. At times I might share part of it with Darrin, but he can't feel what I feel and he is content to let the other two of us get on with life.

The movements of my little friend give me a great sensation of inner comfort and instead of poor sleep, these movements seem to lull me to sleep. I like to feel his feet and bum caressing me from the inside. I find myself chuckling when I imagine that I am getting my whole life's dose of unquestionable love. Once the wee man has been born he will immediately cease to belong solely to me, so at the moment this is my time and I am enjoying it to the full.

I have never really been fazed by all the horror stories of labour, much to every one's surprise, mainly because I have a strong feeling of confidence in my own body and what it can do. All the twinges and odd things I feel tell me my body is just limbering up in readiness for giving me the gift of another life.

Sometimes I find myself saying strange things, because I feel I should. Yesterday someone said to me "Only four weeks to go - not long now - I bet you just want it out." and I found myself replying "Yes, I just want it all over and done with." I was amazed at myself, as this is the exact opposite of what I feel. I would love to have this special closeness with my secret friend for the rest of my life.

I really enjoy my feeling of contentment, of two being as one, and I am looking forward to share this feeling with Darrin and show him what we have achieved together. This is the most important thing that Darrin and I will ever achieve - success in any other way is immaterial and cheap - this is definitely the ultimate goal - this new friend for life for both of us.

* * * * * * * * *

Pregnancy ought to be the ultimate right brain activity. No analysing, no wanting to take yourself apart like a car engine. Instead a total faith in the design of the whole event, a total trust in yourself that your body has the means within itself to look after itself and the growing baby perfectly safely, an enriching satisfying feeling of the joy in the new person that has been created and is developing and an exultant excitement about the fulfilment of delivering this baby in one of the deepest experiences that anyone could ever know. All 'right brain' thoughts, so you can see how you have already learnt how to access your right brain when you have read this paragraph effectively and allowed all the feelings it generates to flood over you. Read it over as often as you need to until you sense how you are getting to your inside feelings and just how good it feels.

This is the kind of thinking, feeling and perceiving that will guide you towards the labour you deserve. Pick this book up and put it down as often as you like and as often as you need to. If you sense that on one day, you're not really getting from it what you want, you're probably thinking 'left brain'. Leave it to another day and run it through again. Read the chapters in whatever order seems right for you - I've just put them in the order that seems right for me.

From your mind's point of view, there is one nice thing about this book - your mind (and especially your subconscious mind) can take it or leave it. If your mind decides this is all a load of cobblers, it will come to that conclusion and you haven't lost anything - you're back where you started. If your mind finds lot of useful bits and links them in with your own thinking, you should realise a considerable element of benefit. If your mind attunes itself to the bulk of the truths that run all the way through this book, there will be every prospect that your labour will be as you would like it to be.

It's fascinating how as adults we tend to approach a challenge with a sense of failure - very much a left brain approach. Kids are spared this - they access their right brain and subconscious so easily and when they come up against a challenge they can just wade in. Watch them play pretend games - you're the shopkeeper, I've come to buy the bread - pouring invisible tea into invisible teacups held by their invisible friends. They want to walk a tightrope or do a backward somersault and they just do it, without any fear of failure. As adults we've nearly lost this ability, and in some ways it's sad. So easily, we approach labour with left brain thoughts and end up with the rotten time we expect.

Yet in pregnancy I can find my right brain and subconscious so easily. I can let my thoughts drift through the events ahead as I want to see them. I sense how normal labour is something I can manage without any more discomfort than it is designed to have. I know in a deep down way that if I let myself trust myself my labour can be all that I want it to be and all that it ought to be - a normal process. As the woman in Whitechapel said all those years ago: "It didn't hurt. It's not meant to, is it?"

Good Childbirth

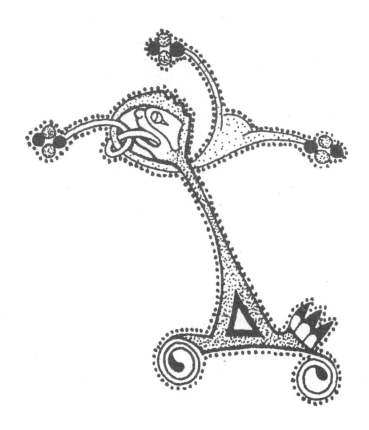

Chapter Six

Let's clear the decks

Have you ever had it happen to you? You've had some guests at a party who are such a pain in the neck that you can't wait to see them depart. With difficulty you manage to shoo them out of the door. What happens next is interesting - instead of just closing the door with a sigh of relief, you stay watching their departing backs until the car drives off. You lock in the quiet exultation that comes with knowing that they really have gone and now you can enjoy the rest of the party. You can do the same with the departing unfavourable imprints. They were there until you took stock and realised how they set the stage for a lousy labour. Now you comprehend how by shedding imprints that are invalid and untrue, you can give yourself a real prospect of your labour being everything you would wish it to be.

As you shoo each imprint out, you can dwell on it for a few seconds and satisfy yourself how untrue and unhelpful each one is. You can satisfy yourself that each imprint doesn't apply to you and that you almost have a feeling of relief as you cast that imprint out. Then you can look at the true and favourable imprints that you can embed in place of the others - helpful imprints that will increase the likelihood of your labour being progressive, manageable and a good experience.

THE UNFAVOURABLE IMPRINTS - ready to depart forever.

1. ***It's bound to hurt, isn't it?***

No it isn't - if it was, it would hurt for everyone. You want to join the happy minority who find their contractions tolerable. You are ready to accept that these contractions are doing their job of stretching up the neck of the womb to prepare the way for that marvellous moment when your baby slides safely down the birth canal that has been formed. If the contractions are really strong, that gives you a chance of making progress more quickly than you ever imagined likely, so your special moment will arrive sooner that you expected. Other women may give themselves those unco-ordinated contractions that do hurt and don't work, but by clearing the unfavourable imprints, you have the prospect of having good co-ordinated contractions that you can absorb.

2. ***I remember the women always scream in films and on television when they are in labour.***

Well what kind of drama would it be if your kind of labour was on the screen? What would make the viewer gasp if all they saw was you getting on with the job in hand, coping with the wave of each good strong contraction as it comes and goes, recharging yourself during the lull and then going along with the next wave knowing that each contraction is one step nearer. We can't blame the film makers, but what they show has nothing to do with what you can achieve.

3. ***My mother told me about the 'pains'.***

You're really sorry to hear what a lousy time she really did have when she delivered you. It's a shame that she wasn't able to clear the decks as you can and that she had a rough time. It doesn't have any bearing on how things can go for you however and there's one great spin-off. When you have an exultant labour, that will give your mother more joy than you can ever imagine. Because she had a bad time, she has secretly dreaded what lay in store for you. And now you've had the kind of labour she didn't even know existed, she is so thrilled for you and you have given her more pleasure than you will ever know.

4. ***My friends told me about the 'pains'.***

However fond you are of your friends, you can distance yourself from them and accept that their experience has no bearing on yours. If they all failed their driving test, does that mean you have to? They all had lousy driving instructors but you have learnt how to drive safely and effectively and when it came to the test you proved it to yourself and the examiner. They all 'learnt' to labour the lousy way, but you've given yourself this breakthrough of learning how to labour the good way, so that when it comes to the day you can labour safely and effectively. Whilst you're sad things went as they did for them, for you everything is a 'whole new ball game' and your labour is a fresh special process of your own.

5. ***What will labour be like?***

You don't know and you won't know until the day. But that doesn't make it scary. You didn't know what getting married was going to be like but instead of being terrified, you were curious, excited and aware of an inner exultation (I hope!!) So why not let labour be the same? In a good labour, there's nothing threatening. However strange these contractions feel, you can trust your body to look after you and your baby and you can trust these contractions to make the progress you need. This has the potential to be one of the greatest days of your life - perhaps the greatest - so let yourself soak up every new feeling that occurs.

6. ***Am I going to burst?***

The simple answer is No, so knowing that, you can trust even the biggest strongest contraction to keep you safe. How strong can your contractions become? Good labour needs good contractions and the stronger they are the sooner you get to your second stage ready for your baby to be born. The further away you can get from really good contractions the less awareness you will have of them, while they will keep on doing their job.

Good Childbirth

These are the brain imprints nearly everyone in the society of today starts with, so assume you have started off with them too. Each one is untrue and without substance. Any of them if retained can set the scene for a lousy labour. They are the main underlying reason why nearly everyone else has a rough time. You are ready to discard them and clear the decks so you can have the good experience in chidbirth you deserve. The text explains how untrue and unhelpful they are. When you have taken on board just why they are not for you, let your gaze wander from imprint to imprint as you satisfy yourself that you have wiped each one out of your thinking. You might see them being cleaned off as if they had been on a blackboard. You might see them disappearing as the balloon around them pops. You might see the balloons with their contents floating away as if someone has cut the string. Or you might just know in an inside way that you have cleared them from your inner thinking and inner brain.

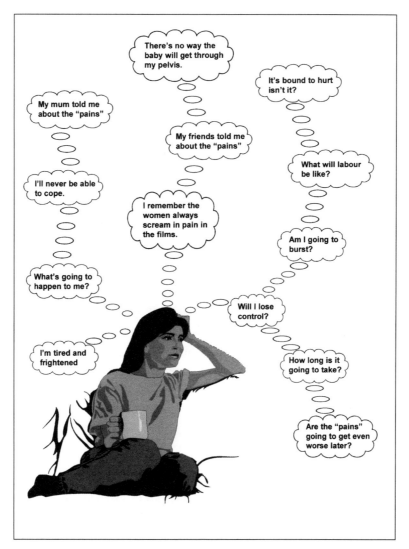

Fig VIII   Unfavourable cerebral imprints

7. *Are the 'pains' going to get even worse later?*

When you remember how perception is the blend of stimulus and experience/emotion, you can see how dangerous an imprint like this is. The language of 'pain' and 'worse' create a momentum of their own. You can let the imprint go but the question behind the question is worth addressing - Are my contractions going to get even stronger near the end of my first stage? A good answer would be "I hope so, because that would tell me that I'm nearly there". And if they do, you know that the mask with the gas and air offers a good way of knocking off the top of those contractions if you need to.

8. *What's going to happen to me?*

Modern obstetrics has in some ways created a monster of its own. It creates the impression that only by its intervention and activities can a woman deliver, and a prelude to that is to hand over herself to the system, whether it be scans at antenatal clinics or epidurals in labour. The woman is left as a regressed infant and feels as helpless as a three year old in a large department store who can't find her mother. Casting away the imprint of losing control, you can instead see modern obstetrics as your ally, coming to your aid if any problem arises, waiting in the wings for the call if it needed, alert to any element of unsatisfactory progress but having to leave you in control of yourself while you continue to progress normally.

9. *Will I lose control?*

This follows on from the last imprint. High tech management can all too easily take control away from the expectant woman. However you have taken stock and realised that modern obstetrics is there to assist you whilst still leaving you to look after yourself in the way that your body is designed to do so. If you allow yourself to trust your ability to absorb all the awareness that goes with contractions however good and strong, then you can sense how there need be no prospect of your losing control. If you are rowing a boat towards the shore when a brisk wind has blown up, you point the boat in the right direction and set your entire mind on making the oars work. You don't stop after every alternate pull and look over your shoulders to see where you are now. You know where you are going and you work on falling into a rhythm of pulling forcefully and effectively, while your gaze might be on the hills on the far side of the lake, that are becoming ever more distant. And before you know it, the boat runs onto the shore and your journey is over. Why not let labour be a similar event?

10. ***I'll never be able to cope.***

If all the imprints you have cast aside were true, then you would have a problem. But every imprint you have discarded has been set aside simply because it is untrue as well as unhelpful. The kind of labour you can have, given good imprints, is one you can cope with far more effectively than you ever thought possible. You can accept good contractions for what they are and by being as far away from them as you need, you can surprise yourself and others by coping more readily than anyone ever imagined likely.

11. ***How long is it going to take?***

Time is but one way of measuring the progress we make. What you are aiming for has been expressed in verse by P J Bailey:

> We live in deeds, not years; in thoughts, not breaths;
> In feelings, not figures on a dial.
> We should count time by heart throbs. He lives most
> Who thinks most - feels the noblest - acts the best.

In real terms you couldn't be bothered if five hours pass or seven. Time distorts in labour anyway and you want to sense its progress more by feelings than by figures on a dial. So you discard the watch and replace it with an awareness that you are getting there and getting nearer to that magic moment everything is working towards.

12. ***I'm tired and I'm frightened.***

It's difficult not to be tired. Sleep for the last few weeks has been elusive - backache, heartburn, waterworks and the baby kicking have all played their part. But frightened is no longer a feeling you need, because you've replaced it with a peculiar inside calmness, a quiet sense of exultation and an inner buzz of exhilaration about what getting to know your new baby is going to be like. To be frightened would make you tense and your labour lousy, but the good feelings you've introduced instead make you peaceful and the prospects of a good labour increase.

13. ***There's no way the baby will get through my pelvis.***

This needs a pretty large act of faith in the the grand design. There's no point in your analysing the matter, but every point in your trusting your body and knowing that all your tissues in your pelvis will move out of the way to let your baby slide safely through. It can work if you let it. Sensing that keeping everything tense will only hold the baby back, you can really let yourself go floppy and slack, so things can make the progress you want.

Now that you've waved these unwelcome guests away, take a quiet look at the picture on page fifty-five. Satisfy yourself that those imprints are no longer resident. If you have any niggly doubts, read through again the text above about the imprint concerned, then look at the picture again. You can repeat this cycle until you sense that you have cleared the decks of all the untrue and unfavourable imprints that in everyone else condemn them to a lousy time.

And now you want to replace the unfavourable imprints with good ones, ones that will support you and strengthen you if the going gets heavy.

THE FAVOURABLE IMPRINTS
- ready to help you look after yourself.

1. *I trust my contractions to do their job on their own.*

You might as well. They'll be far more effective without your getting involved. They are designed to get the job done on their own and all you would do if you did get involved would be to slow them down and make them unco-ordinated. It's a bit like standing over a decorator when he's trying to hang a difficult wallpaper. Once you've satisfied yourself that he has the skill and ability needed, you go off shopping and when you come back, the job is first class. Stand over him and keep on offering helpful suggestions and comments and what happens? He gets rattled, patterns don't match and bubbles appear from nowhere. So you trust your contractions. They know much more about what is needed than you'll ever know.

2. *The more I concentrate on my breathing, the better I'll be able to manage my contractions.*

I don't really know why it works but it does. All you learn at the relaxation classes can come to cushion and help you on the big day. When you use the breathing you have been taught, you find you can get on top of your contractions instead of them getting on top of you. What happens to your nostrils as you breathe in? Just where does the air you draw in get to? How long can you keep it there? What kind of noise does it make as you let it rush out? Go into different aspects of what you feel as you breathe and the longer and more deeply you spend time inside your breathing, the further away your contractions can be and the more they can get on with their job.

3. *Ten good strong contractions are worth more than fifty weak short ones.*

Quite simply, it's true. Weak short contractions hardly stretch and dilate the neck of the womb at all, but good contractions really make progress as the extra dilatation isn't lost by elastic recoil back to the starting position. These are the good contractions you want if you want a labour that gets you to where you want to go.

4. **With a high threshold I can put up with good strong contractions.**

You get a high threshold from your body's own endorphins that dampen down your awareness of the contractions. You get a high threshold by replacing fear with excitement. You get a high threshold by replacing dread with a quiet confidence in your own ability to look after yourself however heavy the going might be. You get a high threshold by clearing the unfavourable imprints and replacing them with good ones. You get a high threshold by knowing you can remain in control of yourself and your feelings all the way through.

5. **The further away from my contractions I am, the less aware of them I am.**

This is an extension of simple observation in ordinary life. Live next door to Old Trafford and every alternate Saturday the noise of a home match deafens you. Live four hundred yards away and you know when it's a home match but that's about it. Live on the other side of town and the only way you find out if it was a home match is to listen to the match reports on the radio. It's the same noise being produced, but the further away you are, the less aware you are. Let the same happen with your contractions. Let them happen, but instead of going down to see what they are like, go off in your mind as far as you choose, keeping as much awareness as you need to let you know you are making progress.

6. **The further away I am from my contractions, the better they will do their job.**

An important concept. You actually help your contractions by leaving them alone to get on with their job. They can do it far better if you keep as far away as you can. So not only do you make yourself less aware of the contractions, but you allow them to become more effective and your labour will progress more swiftly.

7. ***I can spend as much time as I like as far away as I like - my body will keep my baby safe.***

This is a great comfort. You don't need to be with your contractions to look after your baby. Your body will do that safely without you, so you're not needed down there. Everything will be just as safe wherever you are. Whenever you want to, you can satisfy yourself by whatever way you choose that baby is still safe.

8. ***I can't be in two places at once - I'll go off in my mind and leave my contractions to do their job.***

There's plenty of time ahead so you can really go to as many different places as you like and find which is best for you on the day. Happy memories of the recent past or of long ago, perhaps so long ago that you didn't even know that you remembered. Reaching people who may be unreachable in a direct sense and letting them know where you are up to and how you want to share it with them. Looking ahead to the climax of today and to the days that lie ahead. Vividly seeing, hearing and feeling all the dimensions of each experience. And back in the delivery suite your contractions are enjoying getting on with their job. They really don't need you.

9. ***Nobody else knows the half of what I can do.***

It's nothing to do with them anyway. Inside yourself you can give yourself so many rich feelings not only during the rest of your pregnancy but on the day of the delivery. There's a good feeling to be had in a really earthy primitive way and all the feelings are yours - they are nothing to do with anyone else. People seem to forget that labour is a primitive event, not a social event, but that doesn't make it any the worse. It can give you a deep satisfaction that is unlike anything you have ever felt before and it can be very good. You can look after yourself more powerfully than anyone knows. Others just see you on a superficial basis. Only you know the deep knowledge and feelings you have that you can draw on when the going gets tough. It can be a delicious secret to be enjoyed as you hug yourself and your baby in an invisible way.

Good Childbirth

These are the good new brain imprints you want to absorb to replace the rotten ones you've got rid of. These set the scene for your body to look after your labour on its own as it is designed to do. Each one of these has the potential to help you if you can suck it off the page and store it away where you need it deep in your inside thinking. You might work out a way that assists you to take them all on board. You could write them on rice paper and eat them. You could put a slot like a letter box in the top of your head and post them. You could put wings on them and let them flutter to where they are needed. The lovely thing about being imaginative is that you can be as daft as you like and you're the only person who knows. You can do whatever is right for you. Absorb the text that explains how strong and helpful these good imprints are. Gaze at this picture and its messages until you know deep inside that the imprints are where they should be, ready to help you when you need them.

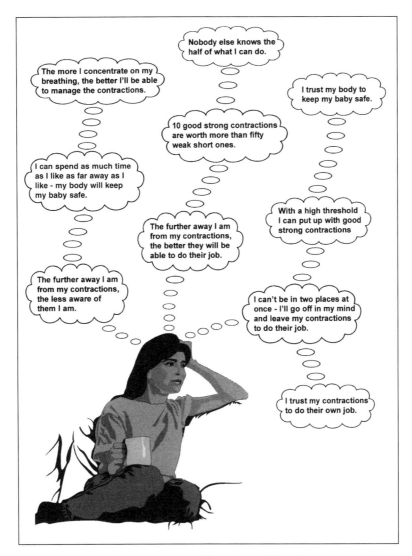

Fig IX   Favourable cerebral imprints

Look at Fig IX which has all these good imprints and satisfy yourself in your inside way that you have latched onto each one and stored it away where you need it. If there are any you sense you're unsure about, why not go back and read over the text that explains it. When you've satisfied yourself that they are all safely on board, let's go on.

You're beginning to sense powers strengths and abilities that you have within yourself. They've always been there unsuspected and now you're learning how to reach them, access them and use them for your own benefit. Illustrations of how women can help themselves resolve problems come in the next chapter in which they tell us how they sorted out their pregnancy vomiting in a way that gives an insight into how you can help yourself in unexpected ways when it comes to going into labour.

Chapter Seven

Puking

When you are throwing up in pregnancy, the last thing you want is someone using dainty expressions like early morning sickness or excessive vomiting in pregnancy. And as for fancy expressions like hyperemesis gravidarum, forget it. It's puking and it's horrible. You feel like death warmed up and dread each day and nobody has the slightest idea how lousy you feel.

What lies behind it? Well, there does seem to be a physical element to it. The woman who is having twins seems to be much more prone to puke than if she were only having the one, even before she discovers she is having twins. For a proportion of women the first indication of a pregnancy is nausea and vomiting, and only then, when they think back and realise they are late, does the thought of pregnancy arise. This suggests that some of the hormones associated with pregnancy trigger the process off. Human chorionic gonadotrophin (HCG) is thought to be responsible. This is the hormone that is measured in pregnancy tests.

On the other hand there seems little doubt that at times a psychological element exists. It seems to be very prevalent in some cultures and yet rare in others. On occasions you feel that the new expectant woman follows the path her own mother went through a generation earlier. The observation that treatment which is psychologically based clears the problem so dramatically suggests that physical factors are the less important part of the cause.

I'm afraid I couldn't really care less what the cause is, because I know the way out of it, even when there is a clearcut physical element.

Inside each one of us is the wish to be famous in some way for some time. In medicine, you could, until about twenty years ago, have an operation named after you, if you devised it. Now operations tend to be given names that describe what is done - a shame really. When I came up with my strategy for clearing pregnancy puking, I thought "Brilliant! Now I'm famous for ever. Reid's strategy is here to stay." We'll have to wait and see.

NLP stands for neurolinguistic programming, which is easy for you to say. It's a typically American over-complicated term for the basically simple concept that lies behind my method. If you're getting a message from deep inside, you go inside yourself and thank whoever is sending that message and tell them you don't need the message any more. There is, as you might expect, a little more to it than that, but that's the general idea.

Later in this chapter you can learn the entire concept. Even if puking isn't your problem, read through the text in a quiet thoughtful way and see what pictures you can produce inside. It's a lovely image to see yourself as an office block and then go down to a little office and go in and see sitting behind a desk a part of you that is you.

When the first three puking women had returned from their journey into their office blocks, I asked each what the version of herself inside the little office looked like. Unprompted each had a similar reply - "Well, I knew it was me, because of the hair or dress, but she had no face." Three on the trot and I was looking at a medical breakthrough.

I thought let's make really sure and a few months later along came another puker. I took her through the sequence and afterwards asked her what the version in the office looked like. Her reply was "I didn't really feel like going into an office, so I got into my swimsuit and swam down inside and then I saw my tiny baby and that she was really there and I knew everything was all right." Needless to say her vomiting stopped that evening. It just goes to show that the patient chooses what means something to her and is usually right. Along came Kathy as patient number five and we were back to 'no face'. I wonder what it means.

* * * * * * * * *

KATHY'S CRIE-DE-COEUR

After twelve years of emotional blackmail and arm twisting, I finally persuaded Nigel that we should try for a second child. Time is a great healer to the memory, yet when I finally did fall pregnant the rose tinted glasses were soon cruelly shattered. I thought I might have got away without it, but at eleven weeks I started with the dreaded nausea and vomiting - the same nausea and vomiting that had haunted me throughout my first pregnancy with Daniel up to the actual day he was delivered.

Immediately the sickness started, the old memories came flooding back. The vomiting got worse each day and soon I couldn't tolerate even the smell of cooking. The look on my son's face when he returned from school to find me clutching the toilet in a passionate embrace each day became so hurtful. I could see he felt so useless and was obviously worried about the wisdom of this so-called happy event that I had painted so enthusiastically.

When the cavalry arrived it came in the shape of my sister who had used hypnotherapy throughout both her pregnancies and labours. During her second pregnancy she had had a prolonged spell of vomiting which I knew she had sorted out with a single session of hypnotherapy. She contacted her family doctor and a session of hypnotherapy was arranged for the next day. It meant travelling over seventy miles, but even if it meant standing on my head drinking tea through a straw, I would have done it. As what was being offered seemed tame by comparison I eagerly agreed.

It was only on the journey to Lytham the next day that I began to question what I was doing. I suddenly realised that I had never really asked my sister what it was about and what would happen. Having to stop a couple of times to be sick helped my resolve, though I could feel reservations beginning to creep over me. As it subsequently turned out I was very glad not to have found out too much in advance, as it made for a fascinating discovery in later conversation with her.

The session began with an informal chat, then I was given a lovely comfortable armchair to relax in. I remember thinking I won't go to sleep if I'm expected to. I felt slightly panicky that I might not be the type of person who would respond to this treatment.

Good Childbirth

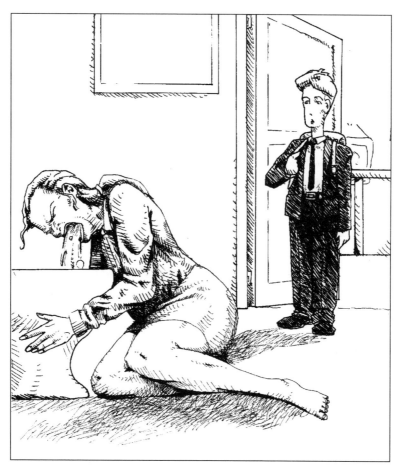

Fig X

My son used to come in from school and find me propped over the toilet bowl

Good Childbirth

Within minutes I could feel myself relaxing so softly that it was almost like melting inside. In my mind's eye I could see myself travelling down flights of stairs, through door after door, down for what seemed to be forever. I felt a feeling of closeness, calmness and a self-embracing feeling like I'd never felt before. When finally I opened the last door, I saw someone familiar, waiting welcomingly - and I realised it was me!

After the session I remember the doctor asked me how I knew it was me and I told him I just knew - I could see the silhouette, the shape, hair, vague features ..... but no face.

That evening I went out to a restaurant I had a huge meal - my first in ages. Later I chatted to my sister alone in the garden. I talked her through what happened and she just listened until I got near the end. As I told her how I opened the last door, we both said in unison "No Face!" This convinced me even more that I was onto something real, as she had purposely not discussed her own experiences with me, which meant that I'd responded from inside with no preconceived ideas about what to expect.

I can honestly say that I was very surprised that the rest of the pregnancy from that day on went like a dream without even a hint of nausea or vomiting ever to appear again. I had a tape recording of my single session which I played occasionally as a precaution, not that it was needed but it helped me relax. In time I gave birth to a lovely little girl, after a wonderful labour and all the earlier arm twisting was worth while.

Now I was back into my 'no face' mode and waiting for the next puker to learn what she would see. When I first saw Helen for the first time at nearly twelve weeks, bag in hand ready to catch the next dollop and looking gaunt, it was 4.40 pm and my surgery was nearly over. I had to be away by 5.30 pm, so we arranged that she would come back after the remaining two patients had been shooed out.

Usually a lot of the preparatory talking is spent in introducing the idea of hypnotherapy and dispelling the common misconceptions that people have picked up from the TV and the press. To save time, it was just as easy and effective not to mention hypnotherapy at all. As you will see, the result was just as emphatic.

Here's what was said to Helen, followed by her account:

What I'd like to do is show you an easy way of finishing with this dreadful vomiting - a way that you will enjoy because it involves your using your imagination, so that when you have rid yourself of the problem, you will be able to pat yourself on the back for what you have achieved.

Whilst you are sitting in this comfortable chair, curious to discover what you can learn, it's important for you to be aware that although puking is grotty, there is nothing wrong with you and more importantly there is nothing wrong with your pregnancy. And just as importantly, after your vomiting has melted away, the pregnancy will still be fine and baby will keep growing safely.

Now for the next few minutes I don't want to talk to 'you' - by that I mean I don't want to talk to the ordinary 'you', the upfront 'you', the 'you' that everyone else talks to. As you may have heard, there is an idea that the ordinary 'you' is in your left part of your brain and is the part of your brain that reasons and analyses things and in many ways does a lot of useful things.

But for the next few minutes I want to talk to a different 'you' - a part of you that is thought to be on the other side, in the right part of your brain. You can consider this the creative 'you', the imaginative 'you', the part that makes instinctive decisions, good decisions, the part that in a deep down way looks after you in a very special way.

And I like to sense that the creative 'you' is your control centre. It sends messages out to other parts of Helen and it receives messages from other parts of Helen. Now at the moment, some other part of Helen is sending up to the creative part a very important message, a very exciting message. You can imagine that the all-of-you is like an office block - lots of different offices with a different part of you in each one, sending messages to each other.

Good Childbirth

But that deep down part doesn't have a very easy or clear way of communicating. It can't talk so it's doing the best it can. This exciting message is that deep down there is a new pregnancy, a new baby has started growing and it's the best news there is. Sadly, the only way that deep down part at present knows of sending up the message is by this dreadful puking.

So what I'd like the creative part to do is to walk down the corridor, perhaps down some stairs, perhaps down in the lift, going past door after door until the creative part has come to the door behind which the deep down part is. And when you've found that door, feel good that you've found it and go gently in. And there behind a desk is that deep down part of you and she's happy to see you.

And you can let her know that you've got the message and you can thank her for that message - even though the way it came through hasn't been pleasant, the news it signified was so very good. You can let her know "message understood". You can let her know that she doesn't need to send you this rather clumsy message anymore, because now she knows that you know. If she wants to send you any message, just to let you know that the pregnancy is safe, she now knows that a warm glow would be a good message to comfort you.

And now that you both know what you need to know and now that you can tell that she is content, you can leave that deep down room and close the door and come back all the way up to where you started from, bringing with you the good feeling that goes with knowing you've achieved what you wanted.

And when you can sense that you are sorted yourself out in the way that you want, you can open your eyes and feel wide awake, interested in what you have learnt felt and experienced and looking forward to enjoying in a special inside way the rest of the pregnancy from today onwards.

There is no doubt that in the waking state this is complete nonsense - by which I mean that it makes no sense to the conscious or waking state mind - and that doesn't matter. To the subconscious it makes perfect sense. If I've got pregnancy puking, my problem is a clumsy message being sent up to me from deep down. I go down and thank the sender for the clumsy message (after all the purpose of the message was to send me good news) and let the sender know I no longer need the message. I satisfy myself that the sender understands and both the sender and I are content. This is what is meant by the concept of trance logic - something that seems without logic to the waking state is full of logic to the subconscious.

If the first time you read the strategy, you find yourself thinking "What a load of nonsense" it probably means that you have read it with your analysing brain or your left brain. Why not go back and read it over, letting your analysing brain go somewhere else? Use your imagination to go into the text. See yourself going down corridors, stairs and lifts. See if you can find a door and be curious about discovering what you find inside. Feel what it feels like - is it brightly lit? - is it warm or cool? - how far down did you have to go?

Once you've let your creative brain or your right brain read the text, you'll feel the difference and be aware that you can sense what lies behind the strategy. It may take a little time and perhaps coming back another day, but it's worth working at it. Learning how to access your creative part is a great gift.

* * * * * * * * *

HONKING HELEN

I hoped when I got over the threatened miscarriage, my problems would be over, but then the 'morning sickness' started. That was when I was eight weeks pregnant and really it was more evening sickness. At first nausea started each afternoon building up to being sick last thing at night, usually when I went to clean my teeth.

Good Childbirth

I could hardly eat anything during the ninth, tenth and eleventh weeks. The vomiting extended earlier and earlier into the day till it included the afternoon and latter part of the morning. The sight and smell of food made me heave and I had to rush to the bathroom.

Sometimes if I sat on the bathroom floor, took deep breaths and concentrated hard on trying to keep down the small amount I had eaten, I could get away with not being properly sick - instead I would just bring up a little watery saliva. Even so I would be really sick at least twice every day, and there was lots of heaving and retching during the rest of the day.

At one point I remember lying on the settee, unable to drink even water. Towards the end of the eleventh week I was taken to the supermarket but after five minutes I had to come out again. The sight of the food was just too much and by now mealtimes were a nightmare. I couldn't face cooking and on the odd occasion that I got the pans out, my husband upstairs in the shower could hear me heaving and crying over the kitchen sink. In fact if it wasn't for the efforts of my family, I don't know what I would have done - as it was I had lost ten pounds in weight.

It was at the beginning of the twelfth week that I went to see the doctor. I think he took pity on me when I went in holding the plastic bag ready to catch the next glup and he asked me to come back at the end of the surgery at 5 pm to learn an 'imagination way' of getting rid of the problem - he told me I wouldn't be sick any more after that.

I was elated but at the same time a bit sceptical. The whole thing sounded a bit like hypnosis to me and when the closest you've been to hypnosis is seeing the crazy things they do in the shows on the television, it makes you wonder. But if it was going to cure me, I didn't care.

I rushed back at 5 pm full of enthusiasm and hope, sat in the chair, closed my eyes as I was told and waited for the magic to happen.

I remember being told that my body was like an office block with different rooms controlling different parts of me.

Good Childbirth

I had trouble picturing at first. I kept thinking surely I shouldn't be remembering all this - perhaps I should be in some form of trance - perhaps I am doing it wrong - but I concentrated hard and there I was walking down a corridor. It could have been a hospital corridor. There were doors leading off and I was the only one there.

I didn't know what 'I' looked like but I remember going into a room and seeing what can only be described as a brain made out of jelly sitting behind a desk. It just seemed to be a big brain, all by itself, floating above a chair. I had to give it a message - something about not needing to send any more messages to be sick. Instead of feeling sick I could feel a warm glow.

I must have come out of that room and suddenly it was all over. It was strange - I hadn't even been asleep. I remember feeling a bit perturbed - was this all there was to it? Where was the swinging watch and all the other things you associate with hypnosis? But I hadn't been hypnotised - I'd just closed my eyes and thought about an office block and a brain. It couldn't work. I felt stupid - brain behind a desk - what would the doctor say!

Perhaps if I got my coat on quickly, I could be out of the door before he asked me any probing questions. Of course he did ask, but he didn't seem surprised when I told him what I'd experienced. What's more, he was so optimistic that he told me I could go back to work in two days time and gave me a final certificate. This was after I had been off for four weeks.

I went home filled with a mixture of hope, positive thinking and total astonishment that that was all there was to it. That evening I wasn't sick - I felt a bit queasy and heaved a couple of times - I kept thinking 'Warm glow'. From then on all I felt was a bit queasy but the vomiting had gone.

I could drink more and eat more and when the Thursday morning came I was able to go back to work. I was amazed. Who would believe that a ten minute session with your eyes closed would literally change your life.

Good Childbirth

Of course the really big change to my life came four weeks later when I had my scan. Here was the reason for feeling so dreadful - I was carrying twins!!

* * * * * * * * *

What is helpful to you is to see how Helen was able to achieve the resolution of her problem without any need for formal hypnotherapy. It is interesting to see that she had a hunch that her imagination treatment was along those lines and this created an element of unease because of the adverse impact made by the television shows. She was able to rise above that unease and sort her problem out completely, even though there was still the twin pregnancy presumably generating huge amounts of whatever hormone is triggering the puking. She found the image of a large jelly of brain floating above a chair a bit weird, but it did the job, so as my third daughter would say "who cares?"

Perhaps the lesson here is that even where there is a physical cause to pregnancy puking, the woman can reframe her body's processes to change herself inside and replace puking with a warm glow. A key phrase I give each woman is to say silently to herself "Other people don't know the half of what I can do." And it's true. Bear in mind that before she learnt to access her own resources, Helen didn't know the half of what she could do.

Good Childbirth

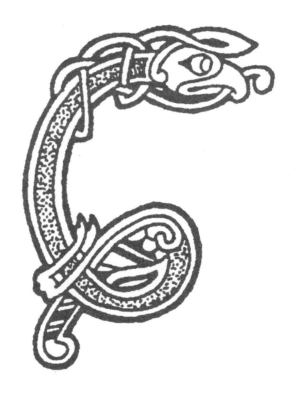

Chapter Eight

Intermission

You're not old enough to remember how trips to the cinema used to be - first the holiday film about New Zealand in garish colour, then the Pathe news and advertisements, then the cartoon and at last the big film. If it was a long film there suddenly appeared on the screen, halfway through the film, the word 'Intermission' came onto the screen and the house lights came up. I never knew if it was to give the projectionist time for a cigarette or to prevent the projector from over-heating.

It gave me a chance to buy an ice-cream from the girl who was able to walk backwards without falling over. Probably the best thing about the intermission was that it gave me chance to find the little blue bag of salt that was hidden near the bottom of the bag of crisps. The other way I found the blue bag was to bite on it and be told by people sitting around me to make less noise as I endeavoured to clear my mouth of a teaspoonful of salt. Great days indeed.

Let's have an intermission in this book - there are three good reasons for doing so. Firstly, if you got this far, you have done some good work comprehending where nearly everyone else goes wrong and working out how you can sort out your own thinking, so that you can pave the way for you to have the labour you deserve. You've earned a rest.

Secondly we can have a look at the remarkable phenomenon of couvade, where the husband experiences symptoms related to the wife's pregnancy - a good example of just one of many mysterious elements of a mysterious process. The application of scientific principles to pregnancy is all very well up to a point, but at the end of the day it must be recognised that pregnancy is an extraordinary event science can explain it up to a point but much remains inexplicable.

Thirdly it gives a piece of Celtic Mythology the opportunity to force its way into this book. One of my earlier books was about a golf course and a section of Celtic mythology found its way into that work, so it has come as no surprise to me that the same has happened in a book about childbirth. And whilst Greek and Norse mythology are in the main heroic, there is a mystical element to the Celtic saga that has a relevance to pregnancy.

COUVADE

This word is derived from a French word meaning brooding or hatching and is applied when the husband experiences symptoms that reflect the wife's pregnancy. We need to distinguish superstitious habits, that seek to transfer symptoms onto the husband, from couvade, where he acquires the symptoms without either him or his wife seeking to achieve such a development.

Superstitions include the beliefs at one time held in Scotland that if the newly wed husband was the first to arise on the morning after the wedding, he would suffer all that went with the labour in subsequent pregnancies and that the midwife could transfer the experience of labour from the wife to the husband by witchcraft. In France and Germany, the husband's clothing was put on the wife to transfer the symptoms of labour to the husband. In the Ga people of Africa, the wife craftily transfers all the woes of pregnancy to her husband by stepping over his body as he sleeps. As a result the Ga men are often lethargic and drowsy while the women are full of energy.

Couvade occurs without it being willed onto the husband. It occurs sporadically in Western cultures and in some developing countries is almost the norm. In the Chagga people of East Africa, the husband can believe he is experiencing fetal movements and in the Wogeo of New Guinea the husband commonly has morning sickness. The Ozarks in Missouri and Arkansas are a culture that seem to have stayed in a time warp and the women say of their pregnancies "My man allus does my pukin' for me."

In the first century AD in Corsica, the expectant mother was quite likely to be ignored while the husband was put to bed and tended for with great care and concern. In some parts of Asia the husband took to bed moaning, while the wife pampered him with food and baths. Upon her delivering, she went back out to work, while he donned her clothing, cared for the newborn and underwent medical treatment including strengthening potions.

Mentioning some examples of couvade shows us how little we really understand of what is going on in pregnancy. While science can analyse many aspects and has achieved remarkable improvements in fetal survival, there is still a deep underlying primitive almost mystical layer that we will never understand, but we can help ourselves by sensing its existence.

If we comprehend how normal labour is a deep rooted primitive process, we can begin to sense why it is best left to manage itself at a subconscious level. By letting the deepest part of your brain look after labour while the conscious you keeps as far away as you can, you give your body a prospect of achieving the efficient labour that is the hallmark of other animals who lack the higher brain functions that we have acquired. When you can trust your primitive and intuitive instincts, you will find that your labour can once again be the dynamic efficient tolerable process it always had the potential to be.

Jacqueline Priya has collected birth traditions from many different cultures in the developing world. She sees the altered state of consciousness that has been touched on earlier and describes it as a state akin to that achieved by shamans and mystics. "It is a time when a woman reaches beyond normal perceptions and may involve a vision of the universe that transcends ordinary reality. It is a time when we go down into the very depth of our being to find the resources to give birth" Having read this far, you will hear an echo of the kind of thinking that you will find helps you so much. To the typical western woman who is unused to moving in these realms of consciousness, this altered state may feel strange, even primitive and scary. But to you it now strikes a chord of familiarity. In pregnancy you have the opportunity to spend as much of your time as you wish enjoying finding your way into this altered state and using it to your own benefit, after you have cleared your subconscious of all the unfavourable imprints that used to be embedded there.

THE CURSE OF MACHA

The tale that comes from Celtic Mythology has been handed down over the centuries and exists in manuscript form since the twelfth century. The usual ingredients of cruelty, violence, sex and revenge make up the backbone of the story.

Many years before Maeve and Cu Chulainn had their great struggles, there was a certain rich Ulster farmer called Crunniuc mac Agnomain who was in great sadness after his wife died. One day a mysterious young woman of great beauty with a shawl drawn around her head entered the house and without a word of explanation fully made herself at home, milking the cows and seeing to the children.

Within a few days she was running the household as though she had been there for years and the children took greatly to her. When night time came she made the ritual right hand turn for good fortune and entered Crunniuc's bed. In time Crunniuc married her and she conceived by him. Her time was to come at the same time as a great feast called Oenach, so she remained at home and he went alone. As he set off, she made him promise never to speak of her in the concourse of men, warning him of the danger that would ensue if he did.

The feast was a great occasion with feasting and drinking and the telling of heroic struggles won and lost. There was dancing and sports and Crunniuc was carried away with the excitement. The main event was the horse racing and when the King's horse won, everyone went wild. The poets started proclaiming verses about the race and when a bystander said "Could anything run faster?" Crunniuc replied "My wife can run faster than the king's horse."

The King was just walking by and when he heard this remark flew into a rage. He had Crunniuc arrested and sent messengers to bring the wife before him to race against his horse. When the wife was brought before the king, she implored him to forget Crunniuc's boastful remarks. "How can I race in the fullness of my child and my time being come?" she pleaded.

Good Childbirth

But the King's heart was set against her and she was ordered to race against the horse. She was dragged to the start and felt the first pangs of her labour. She begged the King not to have her race but he had no mercy within him. He ordered that Crunniuc be brought out and had him beheaded before her.

She turned to the men nearby and implored them to help her, saying: "I am close upon my hour. A mother hath borne each one of you. Plead for just one hour for me and you shall have your race". But the men turned their backs upon her.

"Now, dark woman," commanded the King, "you shall race against my horse, but first you shall tell me your name." Then she cast back the shawl from around her head and drew herself up and her dark eyes blazed with fury.

"I am called Macha, the daughter of Sainrath mac Imbaith, the Stranger, Son of the Ocean. I shall make you and all your people suffer a greater wrong than the wrong you have done me and my man Crunniuc. From this hour the shame you have wrought upon me shall fall on each man of Ulster. This place of the festival Oenach shall ever bear against you my name and the name of that which is within my womb. And until nine generations have been born and have died shall my curse come upon you in times of greatest peril, for ye shall be as weak and helpless as women in childbirth for five days and four nights. Make ready the horses!"

The race was run and Macha in her labour reached the finishing line just ahead of the King's horse. As she crossed the line she swooned and straight away delivered herself of twins, a boy and a girl. As she did so, she gave a great cry and all the men who heard it were enchanted. And the place where she was delivered became known as 'Emain Macha' (the twins of Macha) and was for many years the ancient capital of Ulster. Her curse, which was to last until the time of Furc mac Dallan son of Mainech mac Lugdach, was called 'ces noidhen' meaning the difficulty of childbearing. From the name of Macha also comes the name of the modern city of Armagh.

Good Childbirth

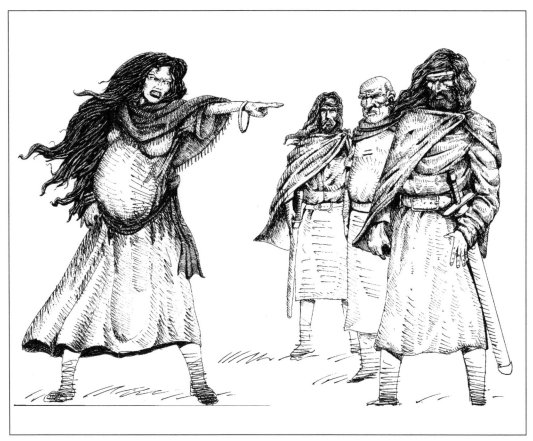

Fig XI

Macha casts her curse on the Men of Ulster who make her race against the King's horse.

Good Childbirth

In each generation that followed every man born in Ulster, once in his lifetime, had to endure five days and four nights of labour during which time he could do nothing and was as weak as a kitten. And never was there more peril than when Queen Maeve marched with her army from Connaught to seize the Brown Bull of Cooley. The legendary hero Cu Chulainn was spared the curse as he was born elsewhere, beyonds the borders of Ulster. He set out to harry her invading army smiting one hundred or more dead each night. Maeve, well known for her scheming, had him agree to meet one of her champions each day at the ford of the river, but he slew each who came forward.

After many days he was getting ever more weary, but then saw striding through the enemy lines but unnoticed by the foe a tall and comely warrior. Instinctively he knew it was his father Lugh of the Long-arm come from the otherworld to assist him. Lugh cast a spell that allowed Cu Chulainn to rest for three days in a trance while Lugh held the ford. The revived Cu Chulainn returned to his post whilst Lugh went for the troops of Ulster, but he found all the grown men under the curse of Macha, unable to stir.

The Boy Corps, the sons of all the Chieftans, came out to battle as best they could but the lives of all were lost. This drove Cu Chulainn into a frenzy and he encircled the host of Maeve in his war chariot. His terrifying shout of wrath was answers by the demons and in their terror the trapped troops stabbed each other in the dark. The scythes of Cu Chulainn's wheels mangled many more and scores of princes and men without number were slain.

* * * * * * * * *

This was the Carnage of Murthemney and ends the telling of the curse of Macha.

Good Childbirth

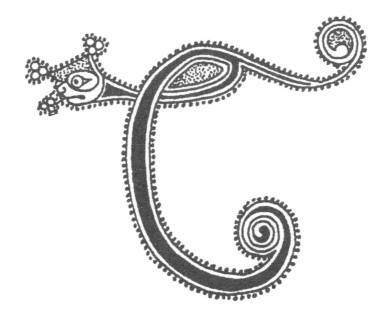

CHAPTER NINE

SO WHERE DO YOU FANCY GOING?

By now it's beginning to dawn on you why all these birth plans and analytical approaches, however well intentioned, seem to fall apart on the big day. It's not just that the woman still has all her unfavourable imprints embedded. It's also because all the preparation and thinking is being done in the left brain, the analytical and conscious part. You can now sense that it's when you begin to do your work in your right brain, the imaginative sub conscious part, that you give yourself a prospect of getting the labour you want and the labour you deserve.

Once you can trust your first stage contractions to do their job on their own, by themselves, as they are beautifully designed to do, then you can realise that the further away from those contractions you are, the less awareness you will have of them. By getting as far away as you can, you will give them a real chance of getting on with their job far more effectively if you are hanging around.

So where do you fancy going? In my early years of working with pregnant women, I used to guide them to options that I thought would help them. The results were indifferent. In the next phase, the women sought to go to the places their conscious minds chose and the results were better. Now they go where their subconscious minds choose and the results are dramatic.

Often they find it quite amusing to have their conscious preference displaced by one that they wouldn't have selected by volition. In a later chapter you will meet Rebecca. In advance she thought she would enjoy once more sun-drenched holidays. On the day itself, she went off into her own kitchen and poured energy into washing pile after pile of dishes!

In this chapter, Joanne gives us a good insight into the strategies women adopt in labour itself and where they go. She was no stranger to hypnotherapy as she had, as a fourteen year old, cleared in a few weeks the masses of unsightly warts on her hands that had refused to resolve in the preceding five years. Now blessed with clear hands she worked at the counter of her bank and had moved away, but when pregnant came back to find out how much help she could give herself by absorbing the principles that are presented in these pages.

JOANNE'S JOYFUL JOURNEYS.

We moved to Yelvertoft when I was thirty weeks pregnant and once the move was done I had a lot of time to practice my hypnotherapy. As a consequence I was able to get into my hypnosis very quickly and easily - it almost became second nature. I used the tape you prepared for me every afternoon and after ten weeks I felt I had prepared myself well for my labour. I remember feeling extremely confident and not a bit apprehensive about the whole thing. I already had a lot of faith in hypnotherapy after using it to clear my warts.

On the Friday evening that Lucy was due, I was conscious that my Braxton-Hicks contractions were becoming more noticeable, but I never considered them to be anything more than Braxton-Hicks. I went to bed as normal and got very frustrated because they were keeping me awake. So as I had done several times during the previous few weeks I used hypnotherapy to get myself to sleep - using that technique you taught me when I came about my warts - going in the lift down and down each floor.

At about four am I woke for my usual nightly trip to the bathroom - pregnancy can be such an inconvenience! - and considered for the first time that what I took to be Braxton-Hicks might be the real thing. Dave was sleeping like a baby (What a stupid phrase - I soon was to learn that babies don't sleep that deeply!) so I left him and came downstairs to time the contractions and have something to eat. The contractions were every ten minutes and although they were getting stronger I couldn't call them painful.

I remember that with each contraction I went into hypnosis and recalled all the memories which I had selected when I came to see you in Lytham. I told myself I was prac-

tising for when my labour really got heavy - meanwhile I kept myself relaxed and occupied with my images as time passed. At six am I lost a little blood so I phoned the hospital who suggested it was time to go in. My contractions were now coming every six or seven minutes but were easily manageable.

I woke Dave and off we went. It took about twenty minutes to get there and by 6.30 we were in the delivery suite. I was examined by the sister on duty and she told me I was nine centimetres dilated. I was absolutely delighted and pleased with how well I was coping with the contractions. I thought to have got to that stage so easily was all down to the hypnotherapy. I remember saying to Dave that if labour was like this I didn't know what all the fuss was about - famous last words!

These contractions carried on for a while and then it was decided that the midwife would break my waters. The contractions after that were a great deal stronger and a lot more difficult to cope with. I remember burying my head into Dave's chest so I could make everything dark and concentrating on my hypnotherapy. I focussed on anything that came to mind. It wasn't my special memories anymore but silly things like counting in my head and visualising the numbers. I also recited nursery rhymes and actually pictured every word. I remember having to block everything out of my mind except the simple images I was focussing on. I was extremely glad when at ten o'clock they said I could push and at twenty past, Lucy arrived.

The hypnotherapy was absolutely brilliant. I was so relaxed at home in my early labour that I am sure that if I hadn't had the slight bleed I wouldn't have got to hospital at all! A lot of my friends were at hospital very early in their labours and spent a lot of time on the ward with nothing to do but dwell on the discomfort of their contractions. Their accounts of their labours and deliveries bore no resemblance to my experience. I also felt that by using hypnotherapy I was actively managing my own labour - I felt I was doing something and that I was in control.

Good Childbirth

The birth of William was a totally different experience. I was induced when I was ten days overdue. From the first contraction to delivery was only one and a half hours. I now realise that I hadn't practiced my hypnotherapy enough to cope with this labour. It was very fast and frantic and the strength of even the first contraction completely took me by surprise. This caused me to panic and I felt unable to cope. I was given a shot of Meptid and I calmed down. Now I found I was able to use my hypnotherapy. This time I concentrated on the sound of my breathing. I focussed on the sound of each breath as I whooshed the air in and out. Soon I knew I was much more relaxed and back in control. The labour passed quickly and William was born extremely swiftly .

The lesson to be learnt from William's birth is that hypnosis doesn't come that easily and has to be worked at. While I was pregnant with Lucy I did spend a great deal of time practising my hypnosis which I did not do while I was carrying William. There is one more virtue of hypnotherapy I must tell you about. It was a great aid in getting back to sleep after the two am feed. All I need now is a course of hypnotherapy to get me back to my pre-pregnancy size!

* * * * * * * * * *

I don't know what she is hankering for at the end as she can be no more that an eight or ten dress size. There are so many good points to lift from her account and you will already have borrowed the ones that will help you. Look again at the strategies that helped her in the greatest part of her first stage and the new strategies she produced towards the end of the first stage, when it was heavy. I liked the transition from the cushion of the rehearsed special memories in to the more basic numbers and nursery rhymes in the dark when the end of the first stage had its crescendo. She didn't need to anticipate or rehearse for this stage - her instincts came up with what was needed.

I thought the second labour was pretty good even if it was different. A short spell of losing control passed, though from the time scale it was unlikely to have been a real pharmacological effect from the injection - that medication will however have been well in the system at the time of delivery and with pethidine could have triggered a flat baby. Listening to the air whooshing was her own tactic she came up with and it worked for her.

As she says, the accounts of her friends' labours bore no resemblance to her experience. Each of them was having a lousy labour while she was having a good labour - you've learnt in these pages the difference. And doesn't it show? I know which one I'd choose.

* * * * * * * * * *

So where do you fancy going? The answer is wherever the creative 'you' wants. Wherever the creative 'you' chooses. Wherever is right for you. In the weeks running up to your labour, put aside some time for yourself. Let yourself daydream about where might be right for you. Go off in your mind and your memories to that place, but don't just snatch a glimpse of it. Go right into your mind and call up all the memories and experiences that go with that place. Spend as long as you like and you need there. Replay getting there and everything you did. Call up pictures of places and people. Hear what sounds there were and what people said to you and what you said to them. Above all feel what those memories mean to you - intense personal private memories that it's good to enjoy once more in the privacy of your own mind.

The more often and the more intensely you can develop this skill before the big day, the more chance there is of your being able to benefit on the day itself and giving yourself a chance of getting as far away from your labour as you want, at the same time retaining enough awareness to reassure you that baby is safe and that you are making progress. You can't be in two places at once, but while 'you' are off in your special memories, the rest of you can stay in the labour ward and get on with making progress. When the second stage comes, 'you' can join the rest of you and really pour all your strength into helping your second stage contractions guide your baby down the birth canal in a powerful and effective way.

All this calls for a huge trust in yourself and your ability to look after yourself. But why shouldn't you trust yourself? You've trusted your body to keep your baby safe all the way through the pregnancy. On the big day there's every reason to trust your subconscious to keep you safe. Look at the ways it looks after you safely already. At a basic level, it speeds up your heart when you run up stairs. At a more sophisticated level, it has guided you in time of crisis and decision making towards selecting the option that was right for you, even though you couldn't explain to a friend why it was the right thing to do.

In the modern era, we have nearly lost sight of the benefits that come from allowing our instincts to guide us and look after us. Those who think they know better than we do would have us analyse and reason our way to the actions we take. In some aspects of life this might be right, but in labour my instincts will look after me far better than reason ever could.

VICKI'S VOYAGE

I woke at 1.30 am feeling restless with a niggling backache so I decided to get up. It was when I was watching television that my first contraction came, though at the time I didn't really twig that this was it. It wasn't painful, just a strange tightening across my tummy. Anyway I thought I'd do some more of my relaxation exercises. I mentally went ahead through the whole process of giving birth. In my mind's eye, I saw myself doing my usual crafty dodge when I got to the hospital. I took all my fears and wrapped them up in a ball, then I locked them away in my bedside locker and left them there. As usual I gave birth to a baby girl.

By 3 am these strange feelings were falling into a pattern of coming and going and it dawned on me that I must be in labour. I locked into my conviction that these contractions were good and that the stronger and more powerful they are, the better. I chuckled to myself when I found myself subconsciously willing them to get stronger and last longer!

Good Childbirth

When it got to 4.30 am and they were coming every five to six minutes I decided to wake David. Being the expert he is, he decided that I wasn't really in labour and told me to go back to bed. It was such a comfort having his wisdom to guide me. I went off and had a bath instead.

By 5.30 am the contractions were getting a little stronger so I phoned the hospital. My contractions were every four minutes so they suggested I came into the hospital. I didn't feel any sense of urgency to get there so I tried to keep as active as possible. I did some housework and then I packed my bag, but by this stage I found I had to stop and lean on something when each contraction came. What I did then was pick out a spot on the wall and focus on it. Then I took myself off to India to a small farmhouse David and I had rented. I sat out on the verandah, doing some washing, watching the sunset across the sea. When the contractions were really strong, the washing got some vigorous scrubbing!

6.30 am and suddenly my thinking changed. I had an irresistible and desperate urge to get to the hospital now so I woke sleeping beauty and he drove me to the maternity unit. I arrived there at 7.45 am and felt my calmness coming back to me. The midwife examined me at 8.30 am and I was really pleased to discover I was 6 cms dilated. She let my waters go and I knew this was really the big journey. They asked me what 'pain relief' I wanted but I knew the gas and air would be all I needed. I was able to focus on my spot and get back to India as often as I wanted.

It was only in the last twenty minutes that I had to stay with my contractions but I wouldn't really say it was painful. All in all I felt everything went as I wanted it to and as I'd practiced a hundred times before. The big shock was just after 10 am when Ben was born and I'd given birth to a boy!!

Good Childbirth

You can see so many good things in Vicki's account and you are probably already picking out the ones that help you. You can sense her poise despite David's helpful advice. She can let time pass and she finds what helps her be as far away as she wants to be. While she's in India her contractions do their job and baby is safe.

Normal labour, which is what she is having, is manageable. She can even do housework. Compare that to your friends who at similar stage - she was probably four or five centimetres dilated by then - are screaming the wall down and ready for their epidural. Her tranquil decision to delay going along with the suggestion that she go into the maternity unit is pretty cool.

So where do you fancy going?

Chapter Ten

The Big Day

There is one simple truth that you should sense in advance - whatever you might think your labour is going to be like, how it will actually turn out will be quite different from whatever you expect. So in some ways it's a waste of time thinking ahead and trying to best guess what it might be like. But what is fruitful is to project yourself ahead and dwell on how you would like your labour to be and how it can be if you just trust yourself and your body.

In the weeks running up to the big day, it is helpful to run through the contents of this chapter in your mind's eye. You might like to read it through quietly, then settle yourself down somewhere quiet and replay what you have read. You might imagine seeing yourself putting a video cassette into the machine and seeing on the television screen the sequence of yourself in labour some time ahead, seeing that you do indeed have the kind of labour that you are working towards and that you deserve, seeing yourself remaining in charge of yourself and your feelings and aware how those there with you are pleasantly impressed with how well you cope.

You might just go off in your mind's eye and go ahead to the big day. Run the sequence of events nice and slowly. Add in your own thoughts to the outline I have set out. Concentrate on not only seeing what happens, but hearing what is going on around you and feeling how you feel inside as progress is made. The more you practice and rehearse this sequence, the more you allow yourself to experience in advance how things can and might be, the more you will increase the chances of your getting the labour you want. Don't ask me how it works, because I don't really understand it, but be prepared to reach within yourself to get what you need.

When the big day does actually come, the first thing you will want to be aware of is the fact that you really have started in labour, that today is going to be one of the most exciting and fulfilling days of your life. It may be that the first thing that will tell you that you have started will be the onset of regular contractions - not the practice ones you have had for the last few weeks, but real ones that you can sense are different. They seem more compelling, more emphatic, perhaps just different. They settle down to coming at regular intervals, so that you can time them. Gradually the interval between contractions shortens and they get stronger and they are lasting longer. At last you can allow yourself to think "Great - today is going to be the big day."

Sometimes the first thing that happens is the waters release first ('my waters have gone') and then after that you start getting good regular contractions, with the interval between contractions gradually shortening and the contractions getting stronger and lasting longer. Whichever way you do start, you'll sense when you are really on the way and feel a buzz of anticipation. You'll contact the hospital and they'll tell you when they want you to attend.

When you arrive at the hospital, you'll know that inevitably there is a fair amount of rigmarole and paperwork to complete, and you won't let it bother you. You'll get to your room and set about discovering what is the most comfortable position for you. You can then settle down to let your first stage contractions do their job. By now you've come to understand that the whole secret in the first stage is to leave those contractions to do that job of stretching the neck of the womb up from whatever dilatation it starts off at, one or two centimetres, all the way up to ten centimetres which is fully dilated. They can do their job on their own, by themselves, without any help from you. The more you can leave them to do that job, the more efficiently and the more quickly they will do it.

What is interesting is that if you did try to get involved with your first stage contractions, if you did try to help them, not only would you do no good, but you would actually make them ineffective. Instead of working forcefully in a co-ordinated way to make brisk progress, the contractions would instead become disorganised and fight against each other - not only would that make little or no progress but they would become painful as well as being useless.

So instead you know you want to leave your first stage contractions to get on with things. They are beautifully designed to do their task, and they can and will make progress if you trust yourself and trust them. You can almost feel yourself becoming a spectator to the wonderful and mysterious process that is unfolding. At the same time, you can choose to retain whatever awareness you want of the progress you are making to reassure yourself that you are getting there and that baby is safe.

But because you trust your contractions, you will know that the further away you get from your contractions, the less awareness you will have. The further away you are from a noise, the less you hear it, although it's still just as loud as it was before. The nearer you go to the noise the louder it seems, though it hasn't changed. And by going nearer you haven't improved the noise - in fact it just annoys you more.

It can be the same with your contractions. By going nearer to them you don't change them (except for the worse!) and you just feel them more. By going further away, you give them a chance to be more effective and dynamic and you feel them less. What you might like to dwell on is where you might like to be instead. We are all different and I'm sure your choice of destination will differ from mine. You will have come across some possibilities in this book but you have probably got better options of your own. It doesn't matter where you go as long as you put a good gap between yourself and your contractions.

Over the years, the women I have worked with have come up with really imaginative ideas. One woman was expecting twins for her second labour. She wanted to go somewhere else, but it was still important to her to know that her babies were safe. Her journey was in a hot air balloon, so she left a cord connected to where she had started from. However far away she was she could still feel down the cord that her labour was still going on and that her babies were safe. I don't know if the psycho-analysts would think this was an anchor to stabilise her or a flashback to an umbilical cord. I couldn't care less. She floated off back to Scotland and found her way back to the village where she had grown up. She let the balloon descend so she was just above the rooftops and could see people she hadn't seen for twenty years. She spent time calling down to them and catching up with their news. Meanwhile back in the labour ward, her contractions did their job and she came back for the second stage. Within a total labour of two hours she was delivered without analgesia of two good sized boys.

You can spend as long as you want wherever you want. You might go off to relive holidays you have had in the past. Don't just flash back for a quick few seconds. Go through the whole event, the airport, the flight, the flat, the beach. Remember what you wore, who you met, where you went for a meal. If you go to the swimming pool, decide what costume you will wear. Look down at your tum and see if you've brought your lump with you or not - some women leave their lumps behind!

If when you've got to wherever you're going, it's somewhere you've been before take some time to recall what you saw, what you heard and most important what you felt when you were there on that previous occasion.

KAREN CRACKS ON

When my blood pressure went up and there was protein in my specimen, I was recommended to have an induction. Shortly after my induction at 7 pm I began to feel fairly good tightenings. Straight away I was offered either an injection of pethidine or an epidural which I thought was a bit odd.

I kicked along till 11 pm without doing very much until the doctor examined me, told me I was just at 2 centimetres and ruptured my waters for me. This got things going in a big way and the contractions really got going, so I used the preparation I'd worked on through my hypnotherapy. David had found the sessions fascinating so he helped me by 'taking me off' to the Maldives where we had been on our honeymoon the year before.

I found it quite easy to go back to that deserted beach, reclining on the sun lounger, the water lapping around my feet, the warm breeze on my face, the palm tress rustling overhead. I went off snorkelling in the shallow brilliantly clear waters, feeling the brightly coloured fish around me, occasionally touching my body. I called out "I've just seen a puffa fish!" The midwife asked what was going on and David couldn't stop laughing.

Shortly after I was giving the entonox some mileage as the contractions were getting heavy. It wasn't easy to prevent myself from going very tense but David talked me through and guided me back to our honeymoon isle.

It was good to sense how confident I felt in myself and in these contractions which I knew were really working for me. On at least two more occasions the midwife suggested I should have an epidural but I knew it wasn't necessary. I gave birth to Bethany at 1.26 am just on entonox and got away without any stitches, so I was very chuffed with myself - and I suppose David didn't do badly.

* * * * * * * * *

Going somewhere else can be funny at times. We will meet Rebecca in Chapter 12, who rehearsed all the good images she was going to draw on when the big day came. When it did, all the practiced images went out of the window and instead she flew off to her kitchen where she washed every dish she had in the house and other dishes she didn't even have. It passed a lot of time in a productive way.

It doesn't matter where you go as long as you get there. Call up different images and see which work for you. Get as far away as you need and spend as long there as you like. What is interesting is that while you are doing this, time passes in a strange 'floaty' kind of way. What might seem to you like quite a short time can be quite a long time and while you have been somewhere else, your contractions have been making progress. When the midwife or doctor examines you, they are often surprised how much progress you have made and it pleases you as well.

Of course in real terms it doesn't matter how long labour takes, as long as you are coping with the contractions and remaining in charge of yourself. It doesn't matter if four hours have passed or if six hours have passed as long as you are making progress and the neck of the womb is being effectively stretched. It hasn't been stretched like this before, and it varies from person to person how readily it lets itself yield. The contractions can take as long as they need and during that time you can float along with them.

Because you are leaving your first stage contractions alone to do their job on their own, you will have reserved all your power and your strength for your second stage, when you will want to get involved. But for your first stage, you just let the contractions come and go, like waves coming onto the shore. Sometimes contractions can be really strong and if yours are very powerful, this should be a development you welcome. It may make them more difficult for you to absorb and cope with, but it gives your labour a great chance of really making progress. Ten good strong co-ordinated contractions can do more stretching than thirty weaker ones. Instead of dreading or resenting good strong contractions, you can help yourself by reminding yourself that these are giving you a real prospect of getting there quicker than you had ever imagined likely.

It is important that you understand that if during your first stage your contractions are so strong that they are hard work to manage, you can do whatever you like and select whatever options you like. Women attending for hypnotherapy have tended to put themselves under pressure they didn't need by feeling that they shouldn't add in other options. I explain that I couldn't care less if on arriving at the labour ward they immediately ask for acupuncture, pethidine and an epidural all together. I'm not on an ego kick and their labour is nothing to do with me, though I do of course wish them well. It's their labour and they can do what they want. What they usually find is that the gas and air ('the mask') is a great help towards the end of the first stage when the contractions often do get pretty steamy.

Over the years quite a proportion have accepted injections of pethidine, and sadly it has to be said this has usually been at the exhortation of the midwife, who has almost insisted the woman has it. It also has to be said that the impact of the pethidine has been consistently disappointing. We'll look at this more in Chapter 13. Let's get back to your labour. You'll remember you were getting towards the end of the first stage.

The last part of the first stage can be pretty hairy as the contractions build up a good head of steam. While they may not be easy to endure, it helps to bear in mind that this crescendo is telling you that you are near the great moment you are looking forward to so much. With the help of those with you and 'the mask' you can forge ahead through this spell until you get to your second stage and get the all clear from the midwives and doctors looking after you that it's now time to push.

Because you have conserved all your strength and power for this stage, because you haven't wasted any energy getting pointlessly involved in your first stage, you will be surprised at just how much effort you can contribute to help your second stage contractions. Because you are in control of yourself and your feelings, you will be able to put so much directed pushing of your own to add to the strong second stage contractions. You'll instinctively know how to push right down into the bottom of your back. The combined forces will help your baby slide briskly and speedily down the birth canal which has been formed by this stage and soon you'll be asked to hold off from pushing and just 'pant'. This is so the passage of the baby's head through your outlet will be a controlled event which is important for the baby and for your outlet tissues. It will be good to continue to remain in control of yourself so you can hold off pushing, however strong the urge might be.

Now at last it is that magic moment you have been waiting for all this time. The baby slides safely out and you can actually see your baby for the first time. You hear for the first time that special shuddering cry that tells you that the baby has arrived safely in the outside world. Now you can touch and feel your baby for the first time and know that everything is all right.

Everything is all right.

Everything is all right.

Lock in to your private memories this marvellous magic moment, one of the greatest moments of your life.

After that it all seems to take place in a bit of a dream. Your afterbirth justs flops out by itself while baby is getting tidied up. You've recognised that at the end of the day it doesn't really matter if you need stitches or not. Even women who get away without stitches on their first baby can be fairly sore from just bruising, so you've decided that you're not going to get bothered if you do need stitches. What does matter to you is how good it is to hear people telling you how well you did and how impressed they were. After you've got sorted out and tidied up, after you've taken the opportunity to hold your baby once again, you can then let yourself have a good satisfying sleep to catch up on the rest you need.

In the days that follow you can enjoy getting to know your baby, this special new person. You can be satisfied about how well you looked after yourself in labour. You can listen to the tales of woe the other women in your ward tell each other and you can silently think to yourself "It didn't need to be like that." You don't want them to become jealous, so you try not to let them know too much of the enriching fulfiling experience you had, but you can see that they are puzzled about the contrast between their labours and yours. Inside you can feel a deep glow.

They don't know the half of what you can do.

Chapter Eleven

What if my labour isn't normal?

By now you must be getting a bit pig sick of hearing about good labour and lousy labour. If it wasn't so crucial, I'd be easing off about it, but as you'll see in this chapter, even when there are factors that mean your labour isn't going to be normal, the quality of the contractions you produce have a large say in determining how things go.

Lynne tells us about her first labour and it sounds as if on that occasion she had the unco-ordinated uterine action story that seems to go hand in hand with the rather intense preparation she had undergone in that pregnancy - the 'analysis and paralysis' phenomenon. She ended up with a section but all was well with the baby, so the outcome was satisfactory in its way. But of course when she came to her second labour, just look at the formula. She was a few days short of her fortieth birthday, on her previous labour she'd only reached 2 centimetres dilatation so her soft tissues had never been stretched and to top it all she had a big scar on her uterus. Any bookmaker would have put odds of '5-1 on' for a repeat section.

LYNNE'S LAST LAUGH

I first became pregnant at the ripe old age of 36. It was a conscious decision with much reading and planning - good diet, low alcohol, off the pill for three months and in the second month of trying I was pregnant. We were delighted and I was only slightly put off at my first hospital visit by the 'elderly primigravida with size three feet - we'll have to look after you!' attitude.

I had an excellent pregnancy apart from a fairly horrendous amniocentesis at 18 weeks. How do you travel to Manchester making sure you have a full bladder for an examination when you don't know how long you'll be waiting when you get there? Near the end I became a chocoholic and my nose was like a tap with catarrh. I started coughing a lot - I was to develop asthma during my second pregnancy.

Tim was away over Christmas helping to nurse a sick father who died at the beginning of January. The baby was due on 6th February and when I went to the antenatal clinic on 8th February I thought they would give me another week. Instead I was told to come in that afternoon for induction. Tim took me in and stayed in with me to see the consultant because we hoped to avoid an induction. When he saw us, he persuaded us to go ahead with a pessary induction that evening.

Early the next morning the contractions started and when I was all wired up I thought I was getting going. Then in the afternoon everything stopped totally and they sent me home for the afternoon and evening with the advice I try a natural induction. Have these people ever tried taking their own advice?

No success and we were both getting cheesed off. On the Sunday morning I went back in and after more pessaries and an enema I was all wired up. There was nothing much doing and I snoozed with the machine on. At about 1 am, the machine went bananas and it was panic stations. I couldn't find out what was going on, but the doors were thrown open and I was rushed down to the delivery suite.

They put me onto a different machine and everyone calmed down as it turned out that there had been something wrong with the first machine. By this time I was getting pretty jittery. My contractions got going but they kept telling me I wasn't dilating. By early evening I was getting tired out and when they broke my waters, things got more and more desperate. They gave me some pethidine but shortly after they decided on a section as both baby and mother were getting distressed. When I came around, no baby! Despite reassurances I was convinced she was dead and I didn't get to see her until the following day.

All in all it was a horrendous experience which I had no wish to repeat. Just about every part of my birth plan had been thrown out of the window and we really felt that it need not have been as bad as it was. When it came to my second pregnancy I was going to be due when I was having my fortieth birthday! I had a good pregnancy apart from the catarrh and coughing. For the last three months I had to keep on getting up to change the giant nappy which I constantly soaked with all the coughing.

We thought about all the options for the delivery. The consultant recommended an elective section but I really wanted to see what I could do. We decided to see what hypnotherapy had to offer because we thought it might give us a chance of some kind of a normal labour.

The hypnotherapy sessions were fine. They were very relaxing and it was good to be able to talk to someone about my fears. However I was very sceptical that it would in fact help me on the day. I was not convinced that anything was happening beyond what I was conscious of, but I couldn't account for the fact that the sessions felt like ten to fifteen minutes even though they lasted for over half an hour. Being able to make my hand so numb that I couldn't feel a needle being pushed through the skin helped me realise that I was achieving something, but I was never entirely convinced that I was 'under'.

The relaxation tapes were wonderful. On the evening of 7th January I used the tape to put myself off to sleep as usual until a coughing fit woke me at 3am. I thought the reason for being soaked was the usual bladder business but as it turned out my waters had broken and soon I could feel I was getting contractions that were quite close. Tim couldn't raise the in-laws on the phone so he had to go and get them and bring them back to look after Chloe. I was pleasantly surprised how calm I kept while I was waiting for him to return.

It was nearly 6 am when I reached the hospital. I did well coping with the contractions, but I had to keep stopping to hold onto the wall between the front door and the deliv-

ery room! When they examined me they told me I was just 2 cms but I felt that this time I was really making progress. They gave me pethidine as soon as I arrived and oxygen because my breathing was a bit tight with my asthma. I settled down to relax and put my stomach at the other end of the room while I just stayed with my head. At 7.15 am they were concerned because the baby's heart was slowing and I was amazed when they examined me and told me I was 8 cm.

By 7.45 am I was fully dilated and at 8.00 am, eleven days before my fortieth birthday, Beth was born, smiling (really!), delivered with the help of Anderson forceps just to lift her out when she was showing signs of distress. I had an episiotomy but the entire experience bore no comparison with the first labour. If it hadn't been for the asthma, it would have been near perfect. If we'd had another baby I would have had hypnotherapy again with you there for the birth, but too late now - as the children say, I've used up all my eggs!!

I suppose my greatest difficulty is that basically I'm a wimp. I seem to have a low pain threshold and worry about everything. Once I get worried, I move into overdrive very quickly and am my own worst enemy. Knowing this doesn't help me do anything about it. The sessions with you in some way or another definitely helped me keep away from pain and the anxiety and I suppose allowed my body get on with it.

* * * * * * * * * *

Lynne will admit that the run up to her first labour was over analytical and intense, complete with the 'birth plan'. Add to this the sequence of failed induction, 'wiring up', nothing doing, sent home, further induction, wonky machine, false alarm, long drawn out non-progressing labour, maternal and fetal distress, caesarean section and baby missing, presumed dead and you can see why the experience was not enriching.

Before her first labour she had gone through the sequence of conscious learning leading to subconscious learning leading to booking unco-ordinated uterine action leading to having a lousy labour. But it's never too late and during her second pregnancy she allowed herself to undergo subconscious unlearning and relearning.

Coming up to her second labour, the prospects of a normal labour and delivery would have appeared to others to be slim. She had however cleared her mind of all the adverse untruths and thus there was now one great weapon on her side - the prospect of producing co-ordinated uterine action. This she managed and she was even able to cope with her husband's disappearance to collect the in-laws before she was then able to have a safe dynamic labour.

From her description we can sense the calm poise and deep joy within her. When the going was a bit heavy, she describes a delightful element of dissociation - "I settled down to relax and put my stomach at the other end of the room while I stayed with my head." This chapter is headed 'What if my labour isn't normal' and while Lynne was at ease, there was some concern in that the waters that were draining were stained with meconium. This means that the baby has emptied bowel content into the waters and often indicates that the baby is distressed.

Compared with the agitation and panic of the first labour, on this occasion a calm monitoring of the fetal heart and sensible use of forceps after Lynne had got to full dilatation and brought the baby's head down her pelvis meant baby wasn't left too long and came out smiling. Credit is due not only to Lynne but also to the staff who helped so well.

To me, this is a good example of a sound balance between the misguided 'let's get back to nature' approach (which has the potential for the sporadic disaster in late labour or delivery) and the wired-up high tech approach which may achieve good statistics but produces a dreadful emotional experience. Here we have a joyful experience in a high-risk but well supervised and managed labour and a safe result.

It is of interest to look at the contrast between the inside Lynne who describes her labour with poise and deep fulfilment and the surface Lynne who describes herself as a bit of a wimp, with a low threshold who worries herself to bits. Her conscious assessment may be right but it shows that it doesn't matter what the surface accessible you is like - the creative inside you is the one who looks after you in the important deep down way.

* * * * * * * * *

The main thrust of this book has been about normal labour. I have looked at the issue from the starting point that things are set fair for a good and normal labour. Given co-ordinated uterine action, that is what you can then have. Set yourself in the unfavourable cerebral pitch and have unco-ordinated uterine action and your chances of a good, dynamic and even enjoyable labour go out of the window.

We have looked at the way we have learnt, in our modern culture, to set the stage for a lousy labour. We have looked at how we can clear the decks, by unlearning in the subconscious all the adverse untruths and relearning all the real truths that set the stage for a good labour.

But what if you have done all this and then on the day there is something in the way things are set that means a normal labour and delivery are very unlikely. Have you wasted your time? Have you in any way given yourself a problem by all the preparation you have given yourself? The answer to both questions is no. Let's see why and how you have still helped yourself.

First let's look at the usual sequence of events in such a situation. Say the baby's head is particularly large or deflexed (which means that instead of the chin being tucked onto the chest, the neck is more straightened). Either of these features can make the labour a struggle. However good the contractions are, the head won't pass through the upper part of the pelvis, the head won't press on the lower segment and cervix and as a consequence the cervix won't dilate.

Until the advent of epidurals, there was a pretty consistent pattern of events. The woman seemed always to have unco-ordinated uterine action and had an awful time. Dose after dose of pethidine was given without effect and she screamed the place down. This was a good move as doctors and midwives paid attention to her. They twigged that she was getting nowhere and she had a section after some twelve hours of labour that had only got her to 2 centimetres. The baby came out somewhat flattened by the pethidine and slept for the first couple of days.

With epidurals, things are better for the woman. She still whacks into unco-ordinated uterine action and now she is given her epidural. She breathes a deep sigh of relief and settles down to read a long book. What happens next is the crunch issue. So long as the staff of the delivery suite are on the ball and keep asking themselves "Is this woman getting anywhere?" all goes well.

She may be lucky and the baby's head flexes or rotates and starts moving down through the pelvis. After the epidural a proportion of labours do seem to convert to co-ordinate uterine action with all the benefits that confers. If these steps happen, she can get to full dilatation and with the probable aid of a vacuum extraction or forceps achieve a better outcome than she would have done in the days before epidurals.

The other option is that she has hour after hour of contractions but makes no progress - the head doesn't come down and the cervix doesn't dilate. This state of affairs can be recognised early rather than late with close care. The Caesarean section the woman is going to end up with anyway can be done before the baby starts getting tired and distressed. Given the vigilant supervision needed, either outcome is a good example of the contribution that epidurals can make in the management of an abnormal situation.

We are not living in a perfect world and there is another sequence of events that can ensue all too easily. In the same situation, the woman needs and gets her epidural. Not only does she switch off but so does everyone else. Staff look in on Mrs Morris, "everything all right, dear?", and move on to the next woman. The crucial question "Are you making progress?" isn't addressed. Mrs Morris can't say as she doesn't know. It's a little to easy to leave her for too long before someone twigs that this woman has no prospect of delivering vaginally and several hours after it became inevitable, she at last has the Caesarean section that she was bound to have and an exhausted baby totters into the world.

What about the woman who has given herself the good cerebral pitch? She comes along with a large deflexed head, but the difference in her case is that she cracks on with good co-ordinated uterine action. With the awareness that is denied the woman who has had an epidural, she can say "Look, I'm having great contractions that are blowing my ears off! Am I making any progress?" Hopefully this will attract close observation and it soon dawns on those looking after her that the head is getting nowhere and neither is the cervix, so let's deliver her before baby gets tired and woman goes through any more slog than she needs to.

When I examined Rebecca at the last antenatal clinic I could sense that here was a head that wasn't going to go through and I put her in the picture that a Caesarean section wouldn't be a surprise - if it was the only practical way of baby being safely delivered, so be it. She was a wee bit miffed having put a lot of effort into her hypnotherapy and coming to labour in a good frame but she heeded what was being said. Let's take up her story.

REBECCA'S ROCKY RIDE

The date I had been given came and went, with false alarms every now and then. It was going to be fourteen days after my due date before I eventually delivered. As the days crawled by, I became more and more desperate to see my baby.

I was frightened about the thought of giving birth, but I kept telling myself there was no going back. Looking on the positive side I was excited about having the baby to hold any day now.

The night before I was due to be induced I had a show so when I got to the hospital the next day I was quietly confident that I would get started without needing an induction. I was getting light contractions every ten minutes but it wasn't anything much so at 11 pm, ten hours after I got to the hospital, I was induced.

By the next morning the contractions were getting a bit more like the real thing and at 9 am they moved me down to the delivery suite. I felt a bit better when Ian arrived to back me up.

Good Childbirth

Only I knew just how scared I felt, not knowing what lay ahead. Somehow even then I didn't really believe that this was happening to me. I felt as if I was dreaming. The contractions were steadily getting stronger and once I was in the delivery suite it was as if someone had turned up a dial. They were really strong and coming closer all the time. One minute I was talking to the midwife and the next minute I had to withdraw into myself, block everything out and concentrate on staying in control.

For a few weeks before the birth I had been attending my doctor for hypnotherapy to help me in my labour. During the first few hours this together with my breathing exercises gave me just enough control to stay on top of my contractions, but when they were right at their peak they were painful. What happened next was funny when my big plan turned itself upside down.

During my sessions and when I was practising at home, I rehearsed how I would use my special relaxation to take me away on beautiful romantic holidays. I was on the beach and by the pool and it was brilliant. When my labour was steaming along, I found that I preferred going somewhere else - off to my kitchen sink! There were huge piles of dishes and the more I washed, the more there seemed to be. I put so much energy into that session at the kitchen sink but even after I had finished more dishes than there were in the whole street my labour hadn't got anywhere. At least when I was in the kitchen I was some way away from those slammers.

From the beginning the baby had been monitored in the usual way, but then they placed an inside monitor, directly on the baby's head. This got me a bit worried as I wondered what the problem was. As well as that it made me uncomfortable as it meant I couldn't leave my bed for the rest of the labour.

I did my best to keep in control by telling myself that the contractions were there to allow my body to help the baby out. By this stage I would be lying if I didn't say they were painful, but by concentrating in myself I was just about able to cope.

Good Childbirth

The midwife was really good and every hour checked the progress of my dilatation. Unfortunately, despite the intense contractions I was making little progress. I got despondent with each assessment and things got to me when after six hours of big contractions they told me the baby's head was tilted and wouldn't come through my pelvis.

I don't know why they left me slamming on for another hour. This got to me as the contractions were unbearable and I could tell that after all the effort I was getting nowhere fast. Then they came along and told me that a section might be necessary, so they were going to give me an epidural so I could be awake during the section if it came to that.

I have to say that the epidural was fantastic. It numbed everything from the contractions and I could talk and think freely. Unfortunately the epidural also slowed the contractions right down, so I was put onto a drip to try and speed them up - it didn't work.

Near the end the baby was beginning to get distressed and I just wanted it to be sorted. They said a section was the answer and gave me a spinal epidural. Within minutes the room was full of people which overwhelmed me a bit. I kept on asking questions and looking for reassurance that the baby was all right. It was a strange feeling - everyone around was so calm and relaxed, while I couldn't stop shaking.

There was no pain and I felt nothing as they delivered our baby boy Jacob weighing in at eight pounds. Even then I couldn't believe it and they could have convinced me that it was a Paul Daniels' trick, that they had brought the baby out from under the table, rather than out of me. I was glad when I looked back that I was awake and that Ian was with me. It would have miffed us if we'd missed the special magic moment.

There are lots of things to learn from Rebecca's story. It's good to be aware that women who have used hypnotherapy to sort out their cerebral pitch and who are going to have good co-ordinated uterine action are still scared at the unknown that lies ahead. Why shouldn't they be?

When the contractions got fairly strong Rebecca withdrew into herself and got on top of her contractions. I know what this means and I don't, but it works. She was still laughing days later at the safe haven her subconscious selected when the going was really heavy. Never mind all this romantic island stuff, I'm off to the kitchen sink to give these dishes a bit of what for!

I can't help but wonder why when they had twigged to the reality that there was no way this big deflexed head was going to progress, that they didn't plump for a Caesarean section there and then. Her contractions had given the head every chance. I mentioned how unco-ordinated uterine action can change to co-ordinated after an epidural, but if you start off with co-ordinated action, the epidural isn't going to augment that.

What is more likely is what happened to Rebecca - the contractions just get flogged and wear out. Drips don't bring them back and the section is now even more overdue. It gets left to the baby to prompt the action needed - he gets a bit distressed and the section that has been asking to be done for several hours is at last undertaken.

Good Childbirth

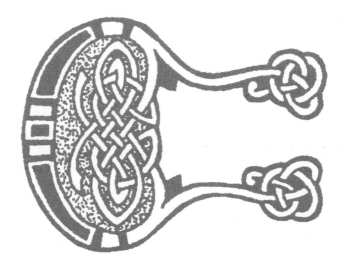

Chapter Twelve

Have we got an attitude problem?

I hope this book will be read as much by doctors and midwives as by expectant women - it is essential that everyone involved comprehends the key to the difference between a good labour and a lousy labour and the way in which the woman's cerebral pitch can play such a large part in determining which type of labour she gets.

I feel it would be true to say that until recent years doctors, both male and female, haven't been a great help in guiding women towards a good labour. Perhaps this is because they are habitually attuned to detecting the abnormal and dealing with it - and simply ensuring that normality is as good as it should be doesn't naturally come top of the list of priorities.

Historically doctors tackled the observation that labouring women were in pain by pharmacological means. The discovery of chloroform and its use by Queen Victoria in labour absorbed doctors' energies for many years. Subsequently medical attention has been directed firstly towards pethidine and related substances and then towards epidurals. Means of increasing the body's natural painkillers by acupuncture and TENS machines have also been introduced with a degree of success.

The initial breakthrough by Grantly Dick-Read and the impetus of Lamaze has enlightened some doctors, but still the dominant medical principle appears to be 'Here is pain - let's diminish or abolish it.' A more far reaching and exciting approach is 'In normal labour I can keep away from painful unco-ordinated uterine action by having co-ordinated uterine action instead - and that I can tolerate.' I would suggest that this is the line you should seek to pursue to have a good labour.

Midwives have probably always viewed labour from a more compassionate viewpoint. The prospect of being able to do much to help a woman who is actually in labour with UUA other than by conventional lines is limited - the woman really needs to have swept away all the adverse imprints before the big day. Midwives must share the frustrations experienced by the women at the drawbacks and ineffectiveness of pethidine. They must be concerned at seeing on occasions babies delivered who have been flattened by pethidine and on delivery forget to breathe. The enthusiasm for epidurals must be tempered by the high incidence of instrumental deliveries and the need for a rather over the top high tech approach to what ought to be a normal event.

When women have reached the labour wards and discussed with the midwives on duty the way in which their preparation has been based on hypnotherapy, the reactions have been varied. In the majority of cases, the midwives have been interested and curious, and have been supportive during the ensuing labour. The demonstrable benefits have been enthused over and subsequently a few of these midwives, in their own pregnancies later, have themselves taken advantage of benefits hypnotherapy can provide.

It has to be said that sometimes however the reaction has been unhelpful. This may reflect scepticism arising from the impression gained from the television programmes based on hypnotic phenomena. It may reflect the commonly held but erroneous view that the hypnotic state involves in some way transferring control of one's self to another, whereas medical hypnotherapy is based on giving the woman more control of herself, her feelings and reactions than she has ever had before. It may reflect the principle "If I can't understand something, I don't like it."

A little nagging thought in the back of my mind wonders about subconscious recall. If I am looking after someone in labour and they are having a good labour, and in my own memory is embedded an imprint of the lousy labour I had, might I feel a sense of baffled jealousy? Not consciously obviously, but is it fair that I never had an experience like this? Perhaps I might be a bit more brusque and dismissive than I should be about the whole matter.

* * * * * * * * *

It is all too easy to underestimate the power that words can have on any of us, at any time. In general medical practice, a consultation can be made or ruined by one sentence. Working with children especially, I can watch them weighing up what they hear and deciding what they make of it and of me. The change in a child when he has to tell what the badge on his jumper means is quite dramatic - he came in with a long face, ready to tell about his poorly ear, but that badge he got for his good drawing was the best thing that happened this week. My ear? Well, that's a bit sore, but it's not as bad as it was. Mrs Cartwright says I'm the best at drawing in my class.

In the hypnotic state, words are often interpreted more literally than usual. A visiting American professor of psychology told me of a consequence of this truth, when he invited a patient to "draw in a deep breath and then expire." The patient nearly bolted out of his chair. The same professor now invites patients to breathe out instead. If you accept my contention that the expectant woman is in a hypnotic state throughout her pregnancy, you will see why I feel words are so important.

When I am in labour, my ears seem to be almost oversensitive to the meaning of words. I pick up meanings that on another day would sail right past me. It's not just that I feel vulnerable - I just seem to pick up more. Bearing that in mind, listen to some of these remarks that can be heard any day in any delivery suite in any hospital:

How often are the pains coming?

Do you want anything for the pains?

Are the pains bad?

We've got pain-killing injections if you want them.

When did the pains start?

What do you want in your birth plan for pain relief?

Good Childbirth

Contrast these remarks with:

How often are the contractions coming?

You're coping really well with the contractions. Do you want any extra help?

These contractions feel good and strong. They should help you make good progress.

If the contractions are so strong that they are difficult to put up with, there are ways we can help - you only have to let us know.

When did you really get going in labour?

What options do you think you might want if your contractions are really strong?

Let's look at how Lisa perceived how she was handled in her two labours.

LISA'S LAMENT

Arrival of Megan 1985.

My first labour was a really good experience though it was harder work than I had expected. My contractions got going at 8 pm and I felt I coped well with them until midnight when Dave took me to the hospital. I told the midwife about the way that the hypnotherapy was proving to be so helpful and she smiled at me in a condescending way and said "Yes, dear."

At 2 am they said I wouldn't be dilated much because it was my first baby. I asked them to check because I could tell that the contractions were strong and productive. Rather reluctantly, the midwife did examine me and was quite startled to find that I was already 7 cm. She changed her tack a bit and I felt quite good as I knew I had got her attention!

I was taken down to the delivery suite and found I was most comfortable lying on the bed. My GP popped in and gave me a hypnotherapy top-up which gave me a good cushion. The midwives didn't seem to understand why he was involved, but when I tried to explain said "You carry on with what you are doing - it's working for you!"

They had told me that the baby was lying very awkwardly and I had a lot of backache and contractions that were very strong. My GP helped a lot and I remember being monitored. I remember the midwives standing around the monitor and they couldn't understand how well I was coping with the contractions. Though it didn't seem long to me, it was 6 am when I was fully dilated and after no pain killers at all, my beautiful 7lb 11oz little girl was born.

Arrival of Matthew 1987

I was ten days over my due date, so I was admitted on the Sunday evening for induction the next morning. They gave me a pessary at 6 am and told me I was 2 cm and to stay on my bed for an hour while I was monitored. I went for a bath at 9 am and while I was in the bath I heard the ward sister say "We will have to slow down the inductions because they are very busy in delivery."

I felt vulnerable and had a good cry. I could feel my contractions but there didn't seem to be much point in my mentioning it - I knew they didn't want me to be ready to go down to the delivery suite. I kept walking up and down the corridor. The other women laughed when I told them I was using my hypnotherapy to cushion my contractions while I was chatting with them.

At 10 am I was just reaching for a cup of coffee when my waters broke. I called the ward sister over and explained that I had been in labour and using hypnotherapy to help myself deal with it. She just looked at me and told me to climb onto the bed, then she turned away and *went off to her office. By now I wanted to push and Dave who had just arrived went down to get her. She waved her hands at him like someone doing voodoo and told him "Tell her to do her hypno thing". He replied "What do you think she's been doing?" When he blew his lid a bit, she did come to me and they put me in a wheelchair straight away.*

I thought I was going to deliver in the lift but I managed to hold on till we got into the delivery suite. Two contractions later and again with no pain killers Matthew was delivered at 10.15 am weighing 7lb 11 oz as well.

* * * * * * * * *

I have been worrying about this chapter which is really for the midwives. I don't want them to feel that they are being criticised but instead I do want to provide an insight into how things seem to the labouring woman. It is useful to know that Lisa is a nurse and two words that would sum her up are pleasant and placid, so the above account isn't down to her winding people up. Talking to many women, I don't feel that experiences like this are out of the ordinary.

Let's go through Lisa's account and pick out a few useful pointers that can show how things could have been better.

FIRST LABOUR

1. "Yes, dear." Does it wind you up being called "dear"? Either use my name or nothing at all. When I am in labour I feel vulnerable enough without being spoken down to or patronised.

2. An old principle - listen to the mother. She feels she might be cracking on and wants to know where she's got up to. Why not examine her first and explain your findings - then midwife and woman will get on fine. If instead you tell the woman she is talking rubbish and then on examining her discover that she was right all the time, she's hardly going to consider you as the fountain of knowledge for the rest of the labour.

3. "I remember the midwives standing around the monitor and they couldn't understand how well I was coping with the contractions." Wouldn't this have been better if Lisa had said "The midwives stood around me while they kept an eye on the monitor. They told me I was doing really well to cope with such strong contractions." Read Lisa's account of her first labour again and you will see that you are probably reading about the type of labour called occipito-posterior that we have talked about before.

SECOND LABOUR

1. "I heard the sister say we will have to slow down the inductions." It's little wonder she felt vulnerable and had a good cry. It's worth giving thought to the impact of overheard remarks. It was probably this remark that set up the pitch for the stages that followed.

2. "She just looked at me" is a very simple statement but it says so much. What a shame the sister didn't say "Well that's a sure sign that you're making progress - are you getting excited?"

3. By now the wheels are coming off somewhat. To tell the husband whose wife is nine minutes away from delivery "Tell her to do her hypno thing" suggests there is a little hostility creeping in!

Good Childbirth

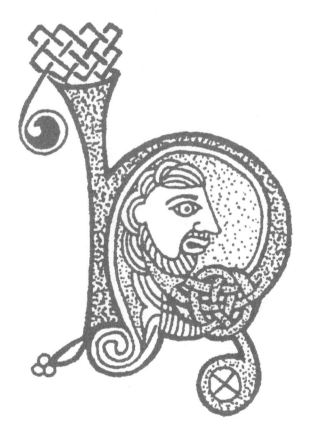

Chapter Thirteen

Options you have for your labour

Let's face it, we're all different and what suits me may not suit you. Some women prefer to have a high tech labour. Given a free choice they would like to be given an epidural just after the second or third contraction, remain blissfully unaware of what was going on thereafter and be pleasantly surprised, on looking up from the magazine they were reading, to learn that they had been delivered of a baby boy. If that was the way your thinking was geared, you wouldn't be reading this book, so perhaps we should look at some of the options open to you that set out to make your labour less uncomfortable.

ENDORPHINS.

The first is the one that your own body has provided, the natural substances that dampens down your awareness of messages that come to your brain from elsewhere in your body. They are called 'endorphins' and the chemicals that have been created in the laboratories as painkillers, such as pethidine, seek to mimic the action of the body's own endorphins.

If something painful happens to you such as breaking your leg, your body produces a flood of endorphins throughout the body to reduce the pain you feel. In late pregnancy and particularly in labour your body produces lots of endorphins, so you experience less of what is going on in your contractions when labour is cracking on. This is one of the powerful ways you help yourself.

There is an injection called naloxone that blocks the effect of endorphins and there have been many interesting studies using naloxone that show how useful your own endorphins are. It has also been shown how using the hypnotic state can push the level of endorphins up, which is just one of the reasons why women who prepare themselves with hypnotherapy have more comfortable labours.

We can look at an example of how this can actually be shown to work in practice. A doctor, whose wife was attending for hypnotherapy, was looking for something which would satisfy his scientifically orientated mind that there really was some substance to this art of hypnotherapy. Now I'm sure you will remember what it feels like if the cuff of the blood pressure machine is blown up way above the level it needs to go to for a blood pressure reading. Some people seem to enjoy whistling it way up. Firstly his wife, while in the ordinary waking state with her eyes closed, let the cuff be inflated until it got to the level she found it hurt - the reading on the machine was 195 - and she indicated this by lifting a finger. Then she transferred herself to the hypnotic state she had learnt to help prepare for her labour and the cuff was blown up once more. She indicated when she experienced the same discomfort but this time the reading was 260.

The level of your circulating endorphins can be higher in labour than at other times, and is increased even more if you have benefited by hypnotherapy or from the preparation you have given yourself in this book. The downside of this is that the endorphin level is lower if you are tired, anxious or frightened - an all too common formula for the woman arriving at the labour ward. The rested, peaceful and quietly confident woman who is ready to trust her body to look after herself and her baby is already halfway to having the labour she is looking for.

ACUPUNCTURE.

I make no claim to have great understanding of how acupuncture might work, but my feeling is that its main effect is through increasing the body's endorphins. If the woman has either given herself a reasonable cerebral pitch or been fortunate enough to have started off with a good cerebral pitch, the labour will be everything she wanted and there have been many such cases reported.

But what if the cerebral pitch is unfavourable, distorted by dread and old wives tales and the laments of others. Two consequences ensue - firstly all the endorphins in the world will struggle to cancel out fear and dread - secondly as we have seen earlier the dreaded unco-ordinated uterine action is more likely and a lousy labour on the cards. I see acupuncture doing what it can from the base of the brain down, but nothing to untangle all the unfavourable imprints that will, if left undisturbed, dominate the labour that is to come.

TENS MACHINES.

Much the same can be said of Tens machines, pulsars and other similar devices that are applied to the skin and probably work in much the same way as acupuncture by pushing up the body's endorphins. They might erect a kind of barrier that dampens down messages on the way up to the brain. All the successes will be in those with a good cerebral pitch and all those who found they still had a tough time will be those whose unfavourable cerebral pitch persisted. Unless the unfavourable cerebral pitch is improved, it is difficult to see how much impact there can be from approaches like Tens machines.

PETHIDINE.

If pethidine worked well and was free from side effects, there would be much to be said from just filling up with it and saying "Take me away". But it doesn't and it isn't. Large studies have shown that it would only appear to be 'satisfactory' in only 22 per cent and in 47 per cent it gave no relief at all. This disappointing degree of benefit has to be set against real drawbacks to the woman and to the baby. Apart from drowsiness and vomiting, a lot of women resent feeling that they are ga-ga and no longer in control of themselves. If there is still a significant amount of pethidine in the system at delivery, the baby can come out zonked by the pethidine and not bother starting breathing until resuscitation and the reversal of the pethidine effect with naloxone save the day. Hardly an auspicious start for baby and a great way of making the woman feel dismay, inadequacy and guilt - roll on postnatal depression.

The particular settings in which the woman struggles, occipito-posterior labours and unco-ordinated uterine action, are the two settings in which pethidine seems to be particularly ineffective, which is a shame. You will have realised that I have little enthusiasm for pethidine and it is a recurring niggle when women are pushed into accepting an injection that they confirm afterwards did so little good. Quite often the reason the woman has steam coming out of her ears is that she is coming towards the end of the first stage and pethidine given at this stage has a real potential to zonk the baby at delivery an hour or so later. By all means have pethidine if you want to - remember it's your labour. But you might like to know how far on the dilatation of your cervix is before you do - often you will be pleasantly surprised to find that you've cracked on and you're beyond the time for pethidine anyway - if I need anything, it's time for 'the mask'.

ENTONOX.

This is the mask, the old faithful 'gas and air', a mixture of oxygen and nitrous oxide, also known as Laughing Gas. I have to pin my colours to the mast here and say I like entonox, if something is needed for contractions that are really good and strong. It doesn't do any harm to the baby and if I am really snorting it, there is more oxygen in the mixture than there is in ordinary air, which can only be good for the baby. I hold the mask so I can control how much entonox I use and I remain in control. If it's making me a bit woozy, I can lift the mask off my face and after a few deep breaths of room air it's all washed out of my system.

The good thing about entonox is that it works - not to the point of abolishing what I can feel but it makes enough difference to help me get back on top of my contractions again so I can tell that I am back in control of myself once more. It meets the conditions I need - it is safe for baby, I am in control of it and of myself, there aren't any significant complications with its use and it doesn't need twenty people standing around me taking over my labour.

EPIDURALS.

I don't want to be seen as knocking epidurals. I think for particular situations and difficulties they have been a major breakthrough and many women in those cases have had good cause to be grateful. For a woman to be able to stay aware for the delivery of her baby by Caesarean section can only enhance the emotional element of the whole event. On the other hand, I feel that for a normal labour an epidural must be considered to be a little over the top.

If I have got my thinking sorted out, I should hope to have a labour that will consist of contractions I can generally cope with, perhaps calling on a little help. To have a needle placed in my back and a cannula left not far from my spinal cord through which chemicals are trickled is getting fairly heavy for what ought to be a normal process.

I can hear all the 'left brains' calling out "What does he know? - he's never been in labour!" At the same time I can hear all the 'right brains' murmuring very gently "Yes - that's true" - and it's them I am listening to and talking to.

My lack of enthusiasm for epidurals for normal labour is based on three main fronts. Firstly, it is pretty high tech - lots of people standing around, monitoring the blood pressure, the contractions and the progress - the woman is tethered like a laboratory animal - she can't move around - the introduction of high tech is in itself anxiety-generating and induces a sense of concern and insecurity. Secondly too many labours have a tendency to need instrumental help. The baby's head often fails to rotate and in addition the woman frequently loses her awareness of the need to push. As a result there is a higher incidence than there ought to be of vacuum extractions, forceps deliveries and manual rotations. Thirdly there is the psychological element. It's all very well to say "I didn't feel a thing" but that loses sight of a huge factor. Childbirth and motherhood are built on feelings - they ought to be emotionally charged occasions - and for the first phase to be void of feelings of any kind seems a bit weird.

There is an awful lot of guff spoken and written about postnatal depression and bonding and related matters. However, the women I have worked with have been consistent for one thing - whether they had a superb labour or were unfortunate to still have a stinker despite their preparation, they have sailed through the postnatal period. Is postnatal depression a consequence of the modern intensive high tech approach? "Give me your labour, - it doesn't belong to you. Let me take away all your feelings." And now four weeks after you are delivered, you are depressed and you don't feel anything. Is it surprising?

Before I dismount from one of my hobby horses, I will set down my perception that the real way to avoid postnatal depression is to have an enriching experience in labour on what should be one of the greatest days in your life. Be yourself in labour and enjoy being in charge of yourself, of achieving what you set out to achieve. Let that magic moment when you have delivered your baby be etched in your memory to stay with you forever, so you can start enjoying the whole experience of getting to know this new human being and becoming the mother you know you can be - and then postnatal depression won't even have a look in.

When Deidre reached the Delivery Suite at 10.30pm on Sunday the first assessment was that though her waters had gone, the contractions she was getting didn't add up to much so she might be looking at Tuesday before she delivered. It came as a nice turn up for the books to be then examined and both Deidre and midwife were pleasantly encouraged to find she'd already got to four centimetres dilatation.

By 2.30am she had reached full dilatation just on gas and air which was great when she was on her first labour and little Martha was about to arrive with a birth weight of just over nine pounds. With a baby that big it wasn't a surprise that the second stage was a slow grind. What is good in Deidre's account is not just the joyfully earthy description of the final minutes but more importantly the exultation and deep fulfilment that burst out of her account of how she feels in the first days of motherhood - it must beat the baby blues any day.

DEIDRE'S DELIGHT

Once I'd got to fully dilated it was a slog. I was pushing for nearly two hours and getting nowhere. The baby's heartbeat was dropping so it was decided the only option was an episiotomy and suck the little bugger out. This stage was really tough going.

Martha Collins was born on the 6th July with the help of a ventouse. She weighed nine pounds and half an ounce and on top of that had her arm across her body and her fist at the side of her face - all these things made the delivery very difficult, but I would go through it all a hundred times just to hold her in my arms.

It was the most magical and wonderful experience. She takes my breath away every time I walk into the room and see her all curled up like a kidney bean.

If you think I sound as high as a kite, just listen to her father!

Good Childbirth

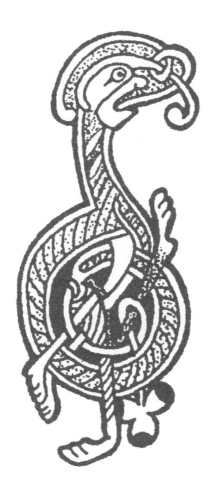

Chapter Fourteen

The way forward

A London taxi driver was telling his friend of the day's events. "I had this fare who was that bloke off the tellie - that Bertrand Russell geezer who knows everythin' about the philosophy of life and all that stuff. So I says to 'im Well what's it all about, this life thing? And do you know what - he couldn't tell me". There are always going to be far more questions about pregnancy and labour than anyone will ever be able to answer. The marvel and mystery of it all is a source of great joy.

It's probably only in the last few hundred years that we in the western world have lost the ability to have good labours. In that short time we have embedded those unfavourable imprints that have condemned so many women to lousy labours. Put into effect the principles we have gone over together in this book and you can give yourself the chance to regain the lost secret of how to give yourself a good labour, how to make progress through efficient contractions that cause you no more discomfort than you are able to tolerate.

It was only in the middle of the seventeenth century that Dunton, travelling in Ireland, glimpsed a population still able to labour well, when he wrote home "And surely if the curse laid upon Eve to bring forth her children in sorrow has missed any of her posterity, it must be here, many of the poorer and labourious sort of women bearing theire children without any long labour or extreame pains as among others, nay without even the assistance of other women, often proveing theire own midwives."

It takes a large amount of trust in yourself to break out of the mould in which today's expectant women are cast. It can be done and when you succeed the exhilaration and fulfilment are immense. You listen to the other delivered women and inside you have a glow knowing what you have spared yourself. They can't understand why you were different to them, why they needed so much help and you needed so little.

Good Childbirth

Some of the maternity units now boast an epidural rate of some sixty percent. Why it should be a cause to boast I know not. Take away the small percentage where it was an indicated procedure and you have a huge number of labours that have been rendered comfortable, but in such a round about way. First give yourself a lousy labour because of your unfavourable imprints, then look for ways of dealing with the bad aspects of such a labour. It's a bit like setting fire to a house, calling in the fire brigade, putting the fire out and calling that a success. My vision is where you don't set fire to the house in the first place. Instead of setting up lousy painful labours and then working out ways of abolishing the painful aspects, why not have a good labour that you can absorb and enjoy?

The octopus of high technology management of labour has its many tentacles firmly wrapped around the women labouring today. The well intentioned interventions are available to you as well if you decide they are for you, but compared with the bright light of a good labour they pale.

What does a good labour feel like? Many women describe a deep seated exhilaration, a sense of achievement and fulfilment. Some feel quite a bit of a 'high' and others a good earthy sense of joy. Later in this chapter, Janet's account gives a good insight into a labour that was progressive, manageable but more than that was, because of her ability to tap into herself, a wonderful experience.

First allow yourself to read what follows next - a trip in your imagination to a place that doesn't exist outside you - in the 'right brain' way of looking at ideas that you've grasped by now. Some women find it helps to make a tape of the text and listen to it slowly unfold. Afterwards bring back from your journey the good things that you instinctively know will help you on the big day.

Time to go to the beach.

> *First see yourself sitting in the middle of a large meadow on a lovely warm summer's day, with the sun shining and a pleasant breeze that makes the clouds in the blue sky move slowly above. As you start walking over towards one side of the meadow, towards the trees over on that side, as you get*

closer to them, it's fascinating to notice that although the leaves on each tree are green, no two greens are quite the same.

But before you get as far as the trees, you come across a small stream, a narrow stream that you could jump across if you wanted to, but it's more interesting to turn and walk alongside the stream, in the same direction that the water is flowing.

And as you look at the water flowing along, you can see the water swirling in little eddies as it slides by - the water is quite clear and you can see down to the bed of the stream. As you keep walking alongside the stream, you can see the stream going into another collection of trees, so as you now are still walking alongside the stream, you find you are in amongst the trees, with the branches overhead intertwined and it's all rather cold and dark. And the going underfoot isn't smooth anymore, as the roots of the trees make the path irregular and it isn't as easy to find your way. And now the water is dark and muddy and you can't see as clearly, but that doesn't really matter, because looking further ahead, you can see that the branches aren't as densely intertwined overhead, chinks of light come through and now you can see the light at the end of the tunnel in the trees.

As you come back out into the open, it's good to feel the sun once more, warming and comforting you and to see that the water is clear once more. And as the stream widens and slows as it flows onto the beach, you can turn away from the stream and leave it as you walk along the beach. If you get rid of your shoes you can feel the sand under your feet and sense how warm it is. You can see the footprints that tell you where you have been and where you have come from. You can hear the waves coming onto the shore and hear the birds and you can see just where you are going. And you can let it feel very good indeed.

And when you come to the end of the beach where the rocks are, you can feel when you rest your hands on the rocks the warmth there. And because this is all in your mind it doesn't seem to come as a surprise to find a door in the rock

- a door that you can work out how to open. Then you can go through the door and enjoy the cool of the inside of the cave in the rock. And on one wall of the cave there are lots of small drawers, just like you've seen on the inside of bank safety deposit rooms in the films. You can decide if you want to put anything away in one of those little drawers, locked away so only you have the key, if you want to. It's up to you.

Then going on deeper into the cave and going around the corner, you come into the most wonderful golden room, a room that almost seems to drip with golden light and it really is brilliant. And sitting there you can see someone special to you who wants to give you their support to help you with the labour that is to come. They may say something to you, or show you something or just communicate to you in a special way how they want everything to go for you in the way that it should and the way that you want it to. You can feel a great sensation of joy and well being from the support they have given you and you can thank them before you turn back to go into the outer cave.

And again you can decide whether or not you want to put something into one of those little locked drawers. Then you can go back through the door, back out onto the beach and feel the warmth of the sun once more. You can retrace your steps, seeing your footprints, going back along the beach until you find your stream, then walk back alongside the stream walking against the way the water flows, back through the tunnel in the trees and back to where you started in the middle of the meadow.

And from there you can come back to where you were before you went away, bringing back with you all the good feelings you want from where ever you have been and aware of the very special inside peace that you have captured just for yourself from your journey and sensing how the encouragement and support you have received is going to help you when the big day comes and when you have your baby.

This journey in your mind can really help give you inner strength and inner peace that will cushion you and guide you when it comes to labour. Janet's account tells how her right brain came up with images and strategies that instinctively helped her have a magical experience in labour. It was not only emotionally rich but progressive - to walk down a flight of stairs a little over half an hour before delivering her first baby suggests that she didn't give the impression to the staff of the hospital that she was getting near the end of the first stage of labour!

JANET AND THE GOLDEN GIRL.

We had decided to end our Easter break with a meal in Lancaster. I was very tired and went to bed at half past nine. At two in the morning I was awoken with a feeling that my waters had broken, but it wasn't very much and I wasn't sure. After a sleepy discussion with David, we decided it was auto-suggestion and that I'd imagined it. An hour later there was a little more leaking but I still wasn't sure. I rang the hospital, packed my bags and checked in at the maternity ward.

I was examined and found I was only one centimetre dilated. I didn't know if it was all a false alarm as I had no contractions I could feel and the monitor showed that baby was fine but nothing else was happening. Dave was sent home and told to phone in the morning. So at six am I was admitted with mixed feelings. I'd feel a fool in the morning if it was all a false alarm. And if it wasn't ....

Once in the ward I got settled into bed with no contractions to speak of and I wondered how I'd cope with the next twelve hours if I was in labour. My plan in the early stages of labour was to use the relaxation techniques I'd gone through in my hypnotherapy sessions, with the pool and the special memories. Depending on how I was coping with the contractions I would be having then, I would look at whatever else was available. My preference was to use as little artificial pain relief as possible but no way was I planning on playing the martyr!

Good Childbirth

I awoke the next morning at about eight. I could feel contractions now but I still managed to doze on and off. I went off to the scenes I'd imagined at my hypnotherapy sessions - being in the meadow on a summer's day, feeling the heat of the sun and looking at the wild flowers, the forest and the distant hills. My dog Barney was with me and we walked alongside the stream.

I remember feeling the first of the strong contractions arriving and I put my foot into the cold water to see if I could distract myself away from them and numb myself with the cold water. I was aware that I was experimenting with options and techniques. This being my first labour I had geared myself up to a twelve hour labour, so I felt I had plenty of time to find out what worked best for me.

I wandered alongside the stream once more and walked the length of the beach, feeling the warm sand under my feet, until I found myself back in my golden room. It was full of people who I was aware had died but who were still very close to me. I was pleased to see my grandparents, my Aunty Amy and a family friend who had died just the week before. I gathered from them the feelings of love, encouragement and support that I felt I needed to get through the next twelve hours or so. I did the trip through the field, along the stream and into the golden room a number of times.

At twenty past ten the nurse came to see me and when I told her the contractions were getting very strong, she asked me to time them and to keep mobile. I couldn't do either! I didn't feel the trip along the river and visiting the golden room was helping enough. I started to think that if I had still had hours to go I wasn't going to be able to cope with all this.

I hadn't really planned exactly how I was going to use the preparation I had from the hypnotherapy but now I knew I had to get the people in the golden room to help me. Why I chose to do what I did next I don't really know but it just felt right at the time. One of my big fears about childbirth was losing control but I could see a way of making sure I didn't.

Good Childbirth

I started to visualise each contraction and then I visualised one big cervix as a huge oval rubbery ring. I positioned myself in the middle of it so I was in the centre of what was going on. My grandmother and grandfather were on one side holding onto ropes attached to one side of the cervix and on the other side with his rope was the family friend who had just died the week before. It all seemed quite sensible.

Each time I felt a contraction it was my job in the centre to keep the environment of the cervix relaxed while they used their ropes to pull it open. There was a dialogue going on between us all the time. They encouraged me to keep the cervix relaxed - they told me how well I was doing when I kept it relaxed and let me know if I was letting it tighten up. They kept me going through really bad contractions and gave me lots of praise when I was keeping the cervix really floppy. I could feel that each contraction was a positive step that was taking me closer to the birth and I could see this big rubbery oval getting bigger and bigger.

By twenty to twelve the contractions were so strong that it was getting too difficult to hold the image of my golden room people. I tried a bath but it was getting too much. The midwife came to see me and by now I had lost my image of my dilated cervix and all the people who had helped me. I thought let's have some analgesia and the stronger the better!

At ten to twelve they helped me walk down from the ward I was in to the delivery suite and I thought to myself how soft I was - I just hadn't been able to do it. On the way down the stairs I had to stop once or twice to hold onto the rail. When I got to the delivery suite they asked me for David's number and rigged up the monitor so I could hear the baby's heart beat.

From the next room I heard the screams of another woman in labour. I remember thinking Oh God that will be me next - I'm just not coping at all. How was I going to get through the next few hours if this all got worse? Someone else came into the room and I thought I hope she's brought some pethidine. She examined me, told me I had done really well and now there was no question of pethidine - it was time to deliver.

My whole body seemed to go into one big wave almost like a convulsion and a desire to push was overwhelming. I was worried I might be pushing too soon but they said I could push, so I did and out popped the head! The mixture of disbelief and relief mingled into one confused emotion. The next push and my daughter was delivered, just as David came into the room at twenty-three minutes past twelve. It was amazing how quickly things had happened - from feeling that it was all too difficult to cope with and walking downstairs to the moment of delivery had only taken thirty-three minutes and from arriving at the delivery suite to delivering had only taken twenty-three minutes.

I was so elated at the way my healthy 6lb 3oz girl had come into the world. I was thrilled how I had done it all myself. The early contractions had been so positive and the people in the golden room had really helped me through my labour.

When I look back at the whole event it was a wonderful positive healthy magical experience that I know hardly anyone else gets a chance to enjoy. Later on when it was quiet and Elizabeth and I were back on the ward, I imagined us both back in the meadow, then walking along the stream into the golden room where I was able to introduce her to the Golden People who had helped me bring her safely into the world.

AFTERWORD

Doubting Thomas was none the worse for being a doubter, but as long as he retained his doubts, he found it difficult to believe. When his doubts disappeared, only then he was able to believe. I imagine there are doubting women who have read up to this point and are saying to themselves "Well, this might all work on a one-to-one session at the surgery, but will it work for me reading this book at home?" I have to say the same thought has hung over me. The reason for writing 'Good Childbirth' is so the message can reach many more women than I can see, but does the message come through in book form?

Shona lives in Edinburgh but had heard of the dramatic transformation in the quality of labour that hypnotherapy could help women achieve. Her family doctor couldn't find anyone in Edinburgh offering help, so when Shona was coming to a wedding down here, she came to the surgery for one chat and session, and then took away a copy of the nearly complete draft of this book. This offered a trial for the hypothesis that because the woman is in and out of a hypnotic state in pregnancy, she could by reading and absorbing the message in the book help herself to a good labour.

SHONA'S SHOWDOWN.

I came to the hospital on the Wednesday with a show and was sent home as I wasn't anything like in labour. I admit it, I panicked! On the Saturday, I had some contractions throughout the day but nothing regular. At 9 pm I had a bath and experienced regular warning signs that my baby was ready to meet me and her Dad.

We came to hospital at midnight and I was a bit disappointed to learn I was only one centimetre dilated. Just before 3 am they were going to send me home, but because I had some protein in my urine I was kept in - Darrin was told to go home but didn't as we both knew Kirtsy was on the way. By 4.45 am I was ten centimetres dilated - much to the midwife's surprise!

Good Childbirth

She then gave me entonox and I was able to last an hour before I had to insist on pushing. I started pushing at 5.45 am and Kirsty was born after four really good pressing feelings - each incorporating me doing impressions of the facial expressions of old man Steptoe (from Steptoe and Son) - I didn't know until then that I could touch my nose with my tongue! I tore a little as she came out so quickly but it didn't matter really.

I'm so pleased that I was able to do all this by myself with no 'pain relief' and I have a daughter who sleeps all night already.

* * * * * * * * * *

This was written the day after delivery and my guess is that Kirsty then settled into the same infuriating habit of waking when it suited her, as my three daughters did. Shona describes what a good labour is like - raw and primitive perhaps, but progressive and manageable - and even enjoyable. Ready to help if they are needed are the midwives and doctors, vigilant and supportive, but when labour is progressing normally, spectators rather than controllers.

Chapter Fifteen

So how was it for you?

It's more of a guess than anything else, but my hunch is that if everyone absorbed all the principles in this book, two thirds of them would have a really good labour and a third would, despite all the great work they had done, still have a lousy labour. This is the overall outcome I've seen in the women I've worked with and reflects the results others have achieved. That's considerably better than any other approach but it's a vexing shortfall and I'm not sure why it should be. There are probably lots of factors at work.

Of course all that it means for the unfortunate third is that they are having the ordinary labour that nearly everyone else who hasn't cleared their unfavourable imprints has, but it's a shame that there is a proportion of those women who have prepared themselves well who do miss out on having a memorable experience.

I hope that you got the pregnancy and labour you deserve. It may well be that during your preparation or your labour your creative thinking came up with some especially useful ideas or images. If so I would enjoy hearing from you with your account and your images. If there is a prospect they would help others, you might find yourself in the next edition!!

My wish is that expectant women find in this book a means of discovering within themselves the gifts and powers that they have always had, but not been able to gain access to. These gifts and powers provide a wonderful cushion against the strife of life and some of the difficult to tolerate aspects of labour. They are a means of remaining in charge of yourself and your feelings. They allow you to experience the good things about labour in a rich and unforgettable way.

Pregnancy and labour - was there ever such a combination of miracle and mystery?

Good Childbirth

Dr Steven Reid
Holland House Medical Centre
29/31 Church Rd
Lytham
Lancashire FY8 5LL
England

About the Author

Steven Reid was born in Lytham where he is now in general medical practice with his four partners. He studied medicine at Trinity Collage Dublin as did his father and brother. After being elected a Foundation Scholar in 1968, he qualified with honours in 1971, being placed first in his year in the Final Medical Examinations.

Before settling in practice he gained extensive experience in hospitals in Dublin and Preston in obstetrics and various surgical specialities, becoming a Fellow of the Royal College of Surgeons of England in 1977.

The work he has done over the last twenty years with expectant women has produced the package of thoughts and ideas behind the book which offers the prospect of regaining the ability to labour in a way that is progressive tolerable and even enjoyable.

He met his wife Mary when she was nursing at Dr Steevens Hospital in Dublin and they have three daughters Siobhán, Helen and Jennifer.

His interests include golf with many years of mixed emotions playing at County Sligo in the west of Ireland and Royal Lytham and St Annes in Lancashire. He had the good fortune to be Captain of Royal Lytham in 1996, the year in which the Open Championship was played there when he presented the famous Claret jug to the winner Tom Lehman.

Good Childbirth

He is the author of 'Get to the Point' a book about County Sligo which combined academic research with lyrical insight into the mystical nature of the course. He has been commissioned to contribute the biography of William St Clair of Roslin for the New Dictionary of National Biography. His prize-winning essay on Misdemeanours in Irish Freemasonry was published in 1989.

This book is the outcome of his quest for new ways of looking at issues, his originality of thought and his aborrhence of conforming to 'the system'. It challenges set views and it is hoped will appeal to searching and imaginative thinkers who want to realise their full potential.

For those who want to analyse and reason it offers little.

For those who are ready to soar it offers much.

Enjoy your great journey.

Steven Reid

Good Childbirth

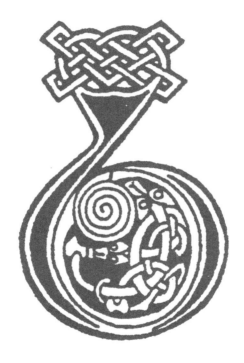

Good Childbirth